Exposition of Ardisia Humilis Vahl in Ameliorating Hepatic Manifestations

Exposition of Ardisia Humilis Vahl in Ameliorating Hepatic Manifestations

By

Biman Bhuyan, Jentinochet Amri and Prakash Rajak

Cambridge Scholars Publishing

Exposition of Ardisia Humilis Vahl in Ameliorating Hepatic Manifestations

By Biman Bhuyan, Jentinochet Amri and Prakash Rajak

This book first published 2024

Cambridge Scholars Publishing

Lady Stephenson Library, Newcastle upon Tyne, NE6 2PA, UK

British Library Cataloguing in Publication Data
A catalogue record for this book is available from the British Library

ISBN (10): 1-5275-5262-4
ISBN (13): 978-1-5275-5262-3

To my students who love and care for nature ....

TABLE OF CONTENTS

ACKNOWLEDGEMENTS

The work presented in this book was carried out as basic research on the standardization of crude plant parts and biological evaluation with special reference to antidiabetic activity based on its traditional usage. During the work, I have received help and assistance from various people, without whom it is not possible to complete my work.

First of all, I would like to recognize the sincere efforts of my student, Mr. Jentinochet Amri, for the painstaking task carried out in conducting the field survey and his tremendous involvement in the various experimental procedures. I express my sincere gratitude to my colleague, Dr. Prakash Rajak, who has contributed in a major way to the compilation, design, and arrangement of the manuscript in a presentable form. I'm indebted to the Department of Pharmaceutical Sciences, Dibrugarh University, Assam, India, for providing the laboratory infrastructure and instrumental as well as chemical requirements for the successful completion of the investigative research work.

I convey my sincerest gratitude to all the faculty members of the Department of Pharmaceutical Sciences, Dibrugarh University, for their valuable help and support during the work. I also express my profound gratitude to my lab assistants, Mr. Bhaben Gogoi and Mr. Pranjal Gogoi, for their help and support during my work.

Last but not least, I convey my heartfelt thanks to Mr. Karuna Gogoi, a traditional practitioner of the village Madhuting, located in the Duliajan area under the Tengakhat block of Dibrugarh district of Assam, India, whose priceless feedback on the traditional usage of various plants in the treatment of various diseases has immensely helped us.

Dr. Biman Bhuyan
Place: Dibrugarh
Dated: 11th of May 2023

BOOK DESCRIPTION

Herbal medicines are fast becoming the default choice for the treatment of diseases. They are gaining widespread popularity due to their general lack of side effects. They are extensively used in the developing world, where, in many places, they offer a more widely available and affordable alternative to synthetic conventional drugs. Most research has focused on clinical and experimental medicine (safety, efficacy, and mechanism of action) and regulatory issues, to the general neglect of public health dimensions.

The book titled "EXPOSITION OF *ARDISIA HUMILIS* VAHL IN AMELIORATING HEPATIC MANIFESTATIONS" is an illustrative account of the usage of *Adrisia humilis* Vahl. in the traditional medicinal system and its subsequent systematic validation and experimental standardization with special emphasis on its prospects in stabilizing hepatic manifestations. It tries to cover the basic aspects regarding phytocomposition, pharmacopoeial standardization, *and in vitro* and *in vivo* studies aimed at verifying its use in the traditional system of medicine. The work embedded in the book successfully upheld the folkloric claims made by traditional practitioners in the treatment of jaundice.

PREFACE

Herbal medicines are fast becoming the default choice for the treatment of diseases. They are gaining widespread popularity due to their general lack of side effects. They are extensively used in the developing world, where, in many places, they offer a more widely available and affordable alternative to synthetic drugs. Most research has focused on clinical and experimental medicine (safety, efficacy, and mechanism of action) and regulatory issues, to the general neglect of public health dimensions. Public health research must consider social, cultural, political, and economic contexts to maximize the contribution of herbal medicine to health care systems globally. Herbal plants or botanical medicines have been traditionally used by herbalists worldwide for the prevention and treatment of liver disease. Considerable studies have been carried out on ethnomedical plants; however, only a few medicinal plants have attracted the interest of scientists to investigate them for a remedy for jaundice.

Assam, one of the biodiversity hotspots, occupies a special place in north-east India. Various medicinal plants for health care are being used for treatments and therapies by village-level healers and practitioners widely in Assam. There are many plants used traditionally for the treatment of liver disorders, but research in this area is still at a primitive stage. The ethnomedicinal documentation, along with the evaluation of the hepatoprotective activity of those plants, may lead to the discovery of new remedies or isolated active compounds.

Ardisia humilis Vahl (Dhsponpoita) is used by traditional healers in the treatment of jaundice and also in fever, diarrhoea, rheumatic arthritis, rheumatism, skin soreness, and vertigo. Roots are used in fever, diarrhoea, and rheumatism, and they have antibacterial activity. Evaluation of hepatoprotective activity will authenticate its traditional use in liver disorders and ensure future scope for this very plant.

The preliminary study involved the evaluation of macroscopic and microscopic characteristics along with the determination of various physicochemical parameters such as ash values and extractive values, in addition to a qualitative analysis of the phytocomponent environment of the plant. Quantitative estimation of phenols and flavonoids was also carried out to add value to the traditional claims.

The effectiveness of the plant in biological systems was successfully analyzed using *in vitro* and *in vivo* methods. To curtail any toxic manifestations that the plant may have, toxicity studies in compliance with OECD guidelines along with histopathological examinations were also done.

The findings of the study were encouraging, as it was successful in backing the claims put forward by traditional healers in the treatment of jaundice.

The entire work has been formatted in the form of a book to enable research workers working in this area to draw on suitable references to carry the work to the next level.

LIST OF TABLES

LIST OF FIGURES

1

INTRODUCTION

BIMAN BHUYAN AND JENTINOCHET AMRI

Medicinal plants play an important role in the development of potent therapeutic agents. Today it is estimated that about 80% of people in developing countries still rely on traditional medicine based largely on species of plants and animals for their primary health care. Herbal medicines are currently in demand and their popularity is increasing day by day. About 500 plants with medicinal use are mentioned in ancient literature and around 800 plants have been used in indigenous systems of medicine.

Herbal drug referred to as plant materials or herbals, involves the whole plants or part of plants, to treat injuries or illnesses (**Winslow & Kroll1 1998, 2192-2199**). Herbal drugs are the use of therapeutic herbs to prevent and treat diseases and ailments or to support health and healing (**Gossell-Williams & West 2006, 217-218**). These drugs or preparations are made from a plant or plants and used for any of such purposes. Herbal drugs are the oldest form of health care known to mankind (**De Smet 1997, 801-840**). World Health Organisation (WHO) has distinct herbal drugs as complete, labeled medicinal products that have vigorous ingredients, aerial or secretive parts of the plant, or other plant material or combinations. The World Health Organisation has precise guidelines for the evaluation of the safety, efficacy, and quality of herbal medicines (**WHO 1991, 1-4**).

The World Health Organisation (WHO) has listed 21,000 plants, which have been used for medicinal purposes around the world. Among these, 2,500 species are found in India, out of which 150 species are used commercially on large scales. India is the largest producer of medicinal herbs and it is called the botanical garden of the world (**Kumar & Kumar 2009, 1-20**).

Herbal drug is a chief constituent in traditional medicine and a common constituent in Ayurvedic, homeopathic, naturopathic, and other medical system. Herbs are usually considered safe since they belong to natural sources (**Rane Jadhao Bakal 2016, 24-36**). The use of herbal drugs due to the toxicity and side effects of allopathic medicines has led to a rapid increase in the number of herbal drug manufacturers. For the past few decades, herbal drugs have been more and more consumed by people with no prescription. These drugs have survived real-world testing and thousands of years of human testing. Some drugs have been discontinued due to their toxicity while others have been modified or combined with additional herbs to counterbalance side effects (**Atmakuri & Dathi 2010, 109-113**).

1.1 Herbal medicine market

As per available records, the herbal medicine market in 1991 in the countries of the European Union was about $ 6 billion (maybe over $20 billion), with Germany accounting for $ 3 billion, France $1.6 billion, and Italy $0.6 billion. Incidentally in Germany and France, herbal extracts are sold as prescription drugs and are covered by national health insurance. In 1996, the US herbal medicine market was about $ 4 billion and the current growth rate may be double by the turn of the century (**Nirali & Shankar 2016, 59-65**). Thus a reasonable guesstimate for the current herbal medicine market worldwide may be around $ 30$ to 60 billion. Global Industry Analysts, Inc. (GIA) announced the release of a comprehensive global report on the Herbal Supplements and Remedies Market. According to GIA, the global herbal supplements and remedies market is projected to reach US$115 billion by 2020, driven by the growing adoption of preventive care as a safe and effective strategy to improve health and well-being. The Indian herbal drug market is about $ 1 billion and the export of herbal crude extracts is about $80 million (**Kamboj 2000, 35-39**).

1.1.1 Overview of herbal medicine

Herbal medicines are a part of Traditional Medicine or alternative or complementary medicine. Herbal medicines are classified as herbs, herbal supplements, herbal preparations, and finished herbal products that contain parts of herbal plants or other herbal plant materials as key ingredients (**Nirali & Shankar 2016, 59-65**). Herbal medicines are extensively used in the developing world, where in many places they offer a more widely available and more affordable alternative to pharmaceutical drugs. Herbal medicine is the use of plants, plant parts, their water or solvent extracts, essential oils, gum, resins, exudates, or other form of advanced products made from plant parts. About 70-80% of the world population, particularly in developing countries rely on non-conventional medicine in their primary healthcare as reported by the World Health Organisation (**Akerele1993, 9-13**). The desire to capture the wisdom of traditional healing systems has led to a resurgence of interest in herbal medicines, particularly in Europe and North America, where herbal products have been incorporated into so-called 'alternative', 'complementary', 'holistic' or 'integrative' medical systems (**Nirali & Shankar 2016, 59-65**).

During the latter part of the twentieth century, increasing interest in self-care resulted in an enormous growth in the popularity of traditional healing modalities, including the use of herbal remedies, this has been particularly true in the USA. Consumers have reported positive attitudes towards these products, in large part because they believe them to be of 'natural' rather than 'synthetic' origin, they believe that such products are more likely to be safe than are drugs, they are considered part of a healthy lifestyle and they can help to avoid unnecessary contact with conventional 'western medicine'(**Awang 1997,341-344**).

A large number of plants and formulations have been claimed to have hepatoprotective activity. Nearly 160 phytoconstituents from 101 plants have been claimed by the Pharmacopoeia Foundation to possess liver-protecting activity. In India, more than 87 plants are used in 33 patented and proprietary multi-ingredient plant formulations (**Roy Das Shil Dutta 2012, 87-99**). Despite the tremendous advances made, no significant and safe Hepatoprotective agents are available in modern therapeutics. For eg. Silymarin is a potent hepatoprotective drug that has established a place in hepatology practice. Silymarin is a flavono-lignan mixture obtained from seeds of *Silybum marianum*. Silymarin is a mixture of silybin, isosilybin, and silychristinanssilydianin. Research on Indian medicinal herbs like *Picrorhiza kurroa* (Kutaki) and *Andrographis paniculata* (Kalmegh) has thrown light on hepatoprotective activity and it is more promising than silymarin (**Kamboj 2000, 35-39**).

1.1.2 Herbal Medicine Scenario in India

The turnover of herbal medicines in India as over-the-counter products, ethical and classical formulations, and home remedies of Ayurveda, Unani, and Siddha systems of medicine is about $1 billion with a meager export of about $80 million **(Vaidya & Thomas 2007, 1-11)**. Psyllium seeds and husk, castor oil, and opium extract alone account for 60% of the exports. 80% of the exports to developed countries are of crude drugs and not finished formulations leading to a low revenue for the country. Thus the export of herbal medicines from India is equivalent to ¾ of its land-exclusive economic zone in the ocean harboring a large variety of flora and fauna, many of them with therapeutic properties. About 1500 plants with medicinal uses are mentioned in ancient texts and around 800 plants have been used in traditional medicine **(Dubey Kumar Tripathi 2004, 37–41).**

The major traditional sector pharma, namely Himalaya, Zandu, Dabur, Hamdard, Maharishi, etc., and modern sector pharma namely Ranbaxy, Lupin, Alembic, etc. are standardizing their herbal formulation by chromatography techniques like TLC/HPLC fingerprinting, etc. There are about 700 firms in the small-scale sector manufacturing traditional medicines with or without standardization. However, none of the pharma has standardized herbal medicine using active compounds as markers linked with confirmation of the bioactivity of herbal drugs in experimental models **(Shi Song Li Yang *et al.* 2014, 78-85).**

1.1.3 Role of WHO in herbal medicine

Two decades ago, the WHO referred to traditional health systems (including herbal medicine) as 'holistic'- 'that a viewing man in his totality within a wide ecological spectrum and emphasizing the view that ill health or disease is brought about by an imbalance or disequilibrium of man in his total ecological system and not only by causative agent and pathogenic evolution, probably implying that the indigenous system drugs (including herbal medicine) restore the imbalanced or disequilibrium leading to the cure of ill health or disease. Such an attitude sent signals that WHO as an organization has failed to provide leadership to establish traditional systems of medicine that provide health care to about 80% of the world population. However, it helped the inclusion of proven traditional remedies in national drug policies and regulatory approvals by developing countries (**Kumar & Kumar 2009, 1-20**). The World Health Assembly continued to debate and adopted a resolution (WHA 42,43) in 1989 that herbal medicine is of great importance to the health of individuals and communities. The redefined definition of traditional medicine thus issued in the early nineties is given by supra. Consequently, in 1991 WHO developed guidelines for the assessment of herbal medicine, and the same were ratified by the 6th International Conference of Drug Regulatory Authorities held in Ottawa in the same year (**WHO 1991, 1-4**).

1.1.4 Herbal medicine standardization

In indigenous/traditional systems of medicine, the drugs used are primarily dispensed as water decoctions or ethanolic extracts. Fresh plant parts, juice, or crude powder are a rarity rather than a rule. Thus medicinal plant parts should be authentic and free from harmful materials like pesticides, heavy metals, microbial or radioactive contamination, etc. The medicinal plant is subjected to a single solvent extraction once or repeatedly, or water decoction as described in ancient texts. The extract should then be checked for indicated biological activity in an experimental animal model. The bioactive extract should be standardized based on active principles or major compounds along with fingerprints. The next important step is the stabilization of the bioactive extract with a minimum shelf-life of over a year. The stabilized bioactive extract should undergo regulatory or limited safety studies in animals. Determination of the probable mode of action will explain the therapeutic profile. The safe and stable herbal extract may be marketed if its therapeutic use is well documented in indigenous systems of medicine, as also argued by WHO (**Kumar & Kumar 2009, 1-20**), (**WHO 1991, 1-4**). A limited clinical trial to establish its therapeutic potential would promote clinical use. The herbal medicines developed in this mode should be dispensed as prescription drugs or even OTC products depending upon disease consideration and under no circumstances as health foods or nutraceuticals (**Kamboj 2000, 35-39**).

1.2 Liver

The liver is a vital organ of vertebrates and some other animals (**Chattopadhyay & Bhattacharyya 2007, 151-156**). In humans, it is located in the upper right quadrant of the abdomen, below the diaphragm. The liver weighs about 1.5 kg and is made up of many lobes called hepatic lobes. Each lobe consists of many lobules called hepatic lobules. The hepatic lobule is the structural and functional unit of the liver. There are about 50,000 to 100,000 lobules in the liver. The lobule is a honeycomb-like structure and it is made up of liver cells called hepatocytes (**Sembulingam & Sembulingam 2010, 89-109**).

The liver is the main metabolic organ in the body. To be able to carry out its metabolic functions, a great part of the blood pumped out by the heart is carried to the liver via the circulatory system. Studies have shown that about 1-1.5 liters of blood are transported to the liver every minute via the portal vein. The hepatic artery brings oxygen-rich blood to the liver while the portal vein transports nutrient-rich blood to the liver. The blood in the portal vein has already passed through the gastrointestinal tract and absorbed large amounts of nutrients (**Ramadori Moriconi Moriconi Dudas 2008, 107-117**).

1.2.1 Functions of Liver

As the main metabolic organ in the body, the liver has many different functions, including:

- Production of protein building blocks (amino acids), proteins (e.g. clotting factors, albumin), Cholesterol and bile acids
- Regulation of the blood sugar level by the production or use of glucose
- Production and supply of bile for digestion of fats
- The neutralization and elimination of waste products of the body's own metabolism and foreign substances such as drugs and environmental toxins
- Storage of nutrients (glycogen and sugar reserves), minerals (e.g. iron), or vitamins (e.g. vitamin B12)
  The liver has also many essential roles in keeping us alive including:
- Blood purification- As the journey of the liver starts throughout the body, the blood from the stomach and intestine is the liver and it prevents the contaminants and also removes the waste products from the body such as; drugs, bacteria, fungi, viruses, parasites, food additives, pesticides and herbicides, chemicals, fats, alcohol, dead cells.
- Detoxification also perform the function of detoxification as it detoxifies alcohol, heavy metal, drugs, chemicals, and toxic by-products from the blood. Housing an ingenious cleaning system, the liver detoxifies infectious organisms, alcohol, heavy metals, drugs, chemicals, toxic by-products, and other poisons from the blood
- Digestion-The liver produces bile, a substance needed to digest and absorb fats. Bile is used in digestion by helping the body absorbs fats and certain vitamins, including vitamin A, D, E, and K.

- Manufacturing- The liver manufactures variable proteins, including enzymes, hormones, blood proteins, clotting factors, and immune factors. The liver also produces cholesterol, which carries energy-supplying fats to the body. Processing- the liver performs most of its function via different organs like skin, mouth, and lungs, Considered to be the biochemical factory of the body, the liver metabolizes substances in the bloodstream.
- Storage- The cells of the liver also act as a powerhouse of the body for many substances, such as iron, vitamins, minerals, and glycogen until they are needed. When blood sugar levels drop and the body needs energy quickly, the liver converts the stored glycogen into glucose and releases it into the bloodstream. In this way, the liver supplies us with fast-acting energy (**Shivananda Julien Godwin Adogwa 2011, 1–5**), (**Akinloye & Moshood 2011, 237-241**).

1.2.2 Liver Disease

Although liver disease is stereotypically linked to alcohol or drugs, the truth is that there are 100 known forms of liver disease caused by a variety of factors affecting everyone from infants to older adults. Cirrhosis is often considered to be a form of liver disease and may be the only liver-related condition that results from permanent damage or scarring of the liver. It is the end stage of many different forms of liver disease and is known to cause several other health problems, including variceal bleeding, ascites, and hepatic encephalopathy (**Sembulingam & Sembulingam 2010, 89-109**).

Many types of liver disease still have unknown causes but the most frequent liver diseases are generally caused by one of the following factors:

- **Viral hepatitis**

Caused by viruses that attack the liver, viral hepatitis comes in many forms. The most common forms worldwide are hepatitis A, B, and C. Although hepatitis A and B can be prevented by vaccines, there is no vaccine for hepatitis C. In Canada, hepatitis C is the leading cause of liver transplants.

- **Alcohol**

Factors such as gender, age, nationality, weight, and health can affect how a person's liver metabolizes alcohol. When the liver has too much alcohol to handle, normal liver function may be interrupted leading to a chemical imbalance. If the liver is required to detoxify alcohol continuously, liver cells may be destroyed or altered resulting in fat deposits (fatty liver) and more seriously, either inflammation (alcoholic hepatitis) or permanent scarring.

- **Genetics**

Several forms of liver disease are caused or thought to be caused, by defective genes. These forms of liver disease may be diagnosed in infancy or may not show up until later in life. Examples include Hemochromatosis, Wilson disease, Tyrosinemia, Alpha 1 Antitrypsin deficiency, and Glycogen Storage disease.

- **Drugs and toxins**

The liver is responsible for processing most of the chemicals and medications that enter your body- this leaves it vulnerable to acute or chronic liver disease caused by chemicals. In some cases, this is a predictable consequence of overexposure or over-consumption of certain chemicals such as acetaminophen or industrial toxins like polyvinyl chloride or carbon tetrachloride. In other cases, chemicals can cause an unpredictable reaction.

- **Autoimmune disorders**

Sometimes a body's immune system may begin to attack the liver or bile ducts causing inflammation and scarring which leads to a progressive form of liver disease. Examples of liver diseases believed to be caused by the immune system are primary biliary cholangitis (PBC), primary sclerosing cholangitis (PSC), and autoimmune hepatitis.

- **Cancer**

Although primary liver cancer is relatively uncommon, many other forms of cancer often metastasize in the liver. Because the liver filters a high volume of blood which may be carrying cancer cells, it is susceptible to developing a form of secondary cancer. If cancer originates in the liver, it is often caused by hepatitis B and hepatitis C or it can develop in cases of advanced liver disease when cirrhosis is present (**Sembulingam & Sembulingam 2010, 89-109**).

1.2.3 Signs and Symptoms of liver disease

Although the difference in signs and symptoms can vary so much from one drug to the next, and one patient to the next some common signs associated with drug-induced hepatotoxicity include; Non-specific symptoms: ones that may not directly pinpoint the problem.

- Fatigue
- Abdominal pain and swelling.
- Weakness
- Loss of appetite

Signs and symptoms specific for hepatotoxicity-

- Jaundice
- Itching
- Easily bruising

When the liver is severely damaged cirrhosis can occur. Symptoms of cirrhosis include

- Edema (oftentimes in the legs)
- Mental confusion
- Kidney failure
- Gastrointestinal bleeding
- Vulnerability to bacterial infection

Accumulated toxins in the body place a constant drag on the immune system, setting the stage for autoimmune diseases and cancer. If any organ is compromised, others will be affected, eventually leading to a cumulative negative effect on health. Some of the most toxic legal substances people flood their livers with are alcohol and medication. Alcohol- acetaldehyde is a highly toxic substance obtained from the metabolism of alcohol is the molecule that causes impairment or drunkenness. Scientists have discovered that when acetaldehyde is bound to human liver plasma membranes, liver cells die (**Rane Jadhao Bakal 2016, 24-36**).

1.2.4 Drug-Induced Hepatotoxicity

Two drugs (Bromfenac and troglitazone) have been withdrawn from the market by the Food and Drug Administration (FDA) for causing severe liver injury, a potential danger that had not been fully recognized in the course of the preapproval clinical trials. Reports of adverse drug reactions of any type engender fear and skepticism in the public about the actions of the pharmaceutical industry and the FDA (**Lazarou Bruce Paul 1998, 1200-1205**). Drug-induced hepatic injury is the most frequent reason for the withdrawal from the market of an approved drug, and it also accounts for more than 50 percent of the cause of acute liver failure in the United States today. More than 75 percent of the case of idiosyncratic drug reactions results in liver transplantation or death (**Ostapowicz Fontana Schiødt Larson *et al.*2002, 947-954**). Recent efforts by the National Institute of Health and the FDA have been directed toward a better understanding of these occurrences to improve the outcomes (**Bissell Montgomery Gregory Debra *et al.* 2001, 1009-1013**), (**Weber Meinrad Stampfl 2003, 105-136**).

1.2.5 Mechanism

In some physiological conditions, the mitochondrial membrane can lose its structure and functional integrity by the opening of the mitochondrial permeability transitional pore (MPTP) and this can disturb ATP synthesis and storage. Impaired ATP synthesis causes a sudden increase in Intracellular calcium levels by the activation of plasma membrane calcium ATPase (PMCA (**Wallace Weiwei Procaccio2010, 297**). Sometimes MPTP opening also allows the release of proteins, such as caspases, Cytochrome C, and Apoptosis-inducing factor (**Masubuchi Chieko Toshiharu 2005, 110-116**), (**Pessayre Abdellah Berson Fromenty 2010, 311-365**). These components can bind with the Apaf protein leading to initiating the apoptosis pathway through caspase 9 and caspase 3 activation (**Fulda Lorenzo Guido 2010, 447-464**), (**Pessayre Delphine Fau Marie *et al.*1999, 760-770**). MPTM opening is mostly induced by several drugs, xenobiotics, or some endogenous by-products like calcium, and fatty acid of bile salt **(Malhi Gregory Lemasters 2006, S31-S44)**. Mitochondria produce Reactive Oxygen species (ROS) via the activity of the Mitochondrial Respiratory chain (MRC) (**Seifert Carmen Jian Harper 2010, 5748-5758**). In normal cases, ROS can be detoxified through glutathione peroxidase (GPx) using glutathione as a cofactor. Depletion in GSH causes H2O2 accumulation and this whole process turns out as MPTP opening, JNK (c-Jun N-terminal kinase) activation, and activation of p38 HSP22 apoptotic pathway **(Fernandez Ritter Wendell Linehan *et al.* 2005, 845-853)**, **(Jones Lemasters Derick Urs *et. al.* 2010, 98)**. This High level of ROS can also damage oxidative phosphorylation protein (OXPOS), cardiolipin, and mitochondrial DNA which leads to cytosolic hepatitis (**Demeilliers Caroline Alain Abdellah *et al.* 2002, 1278-1290**), (**Sanz Pilar Victoria Manuel *et. al.*2006, 1064-1073**), (**Velsor Kovacevic Kovacevic Leitner *et. al.*2004, 10-19**). Drugs, exogenous compounds, ethanol assumption, fasting, and several viral diseases have the ability of GSH depletion (**Fromenty Igoudjil Pessayre 2004, 121-138**). Some drugs and ethanol intoxication can also inhibit mitochondrial beta-oxidation that can lead to microvesicular steatosis in the form of triglycerides accumulation in hepatocytes (**Coghlan Sommadossi Jhala Many *et al.*2001,1914-1921**), (**Danan Bernuau Jacques Claude *et al.*1985, 210-213**), (**Kleiner Gaffey Sallie Tsokos *et al.*1997, 192-199**). These triglycerides are found in the form of various cytoplasmic lipid droplets that can be stained by oil red (**Hautekeete & Benhamou1990, 311-326**), (**Le Bricquir Dominique Pierre Georges *et al.*1994, 771-773**). Large amounts of lipid accumulation in hepatocytes can cause macrovascular steatosis (Steatohepatitis) which is also known as Fatty liver. Drugs like tamoxifen, TZDs, irinotecan, and perhexiline induce non-alcoholic fatty liver disease (NAFLD) in obese and diabetic patients (**Bruno Patrick Paola Nicole *et al.*2005, 932**), (**Ruiz Rodríguez-Juan Teresa Martínez *et al.* 2007, 414-423**), (**Rosenberg Johannesson Ros Lindholm 2007, 1111-1118**). A recent case shows that Insulin resistance and hyperinsulinemia can also induce hepatic liver injury (**Saphner Shirley Hailun Paul 2009, 3189-3195**), (**Begriche Laetitia Julie Marie-Anne *et al.*2009, e11-e23**), (**Fabbrini Shelby Samuel 2010, 679-689**). Some antipsychotic drugs can also increase food intake thus leading to obesity via the mechanism of disruption of leptin signaling or 5-HT2c serotoninergic receptor. Antipsychotic drugs may also trigger lipogenesis in hepatocytes and adipose tissue through activation of SREBP (Sterol regulatory element- binding protein) (**Cahill Carol Masayuki Hiromasa *et al.*2002, 907-915**), (**Lauressergues Bart Karine Zouher *et al.* 2010, 427-439**), (**Yang Tzer Sung Yen 2007, 202-208**).

1.3 Hepatotoxic Agents

CCl_4 Induced Hepatotoxicity

Carbon tetrachloride (CCl_4) induced liver damage has been lengthily used as an experimental model. CCl_4 is used as a model drug for the study of hepatotoxicity in acute and chronic liver failure. CCl_4 is metabolized by CYP2E1, CYP2B and possibly CYP3A to form the trichloromethyl radical, CCl_3. This CCl_3 can also bind to cellular molecules damaging crucial cellular progressions. This radical can also react with oxygen to form the trichloromethylperoxy radical CCl3OO, a highly reactive species. The metabolites of CCl_4 cause hepatic injury in the CCl_4 acute liver injury model (**Weber Meinrad Stampfl 2003, 105-136**). Administration of a single dose of CCl_4 to rats produces centrilobular necrosis and fatty changes. The poison reaches its maximum concentration in the liver within 3 hours of administration. Afterwards, the level falls and by 24 hours there is no CCl_4 left in the liver. Dose of CCl_4: 0.1 to 3ml/kg I.P (**Dawkins 1963, 189-196).**

Galactosamine Induced Hepatoxicity

Galactosamine is hepatotoxin generally used as a hepatotoxic compound. D-Galactosamine a discerning hepatotoxic, induces a verbose type of liver injury closely like human biological hepatitis and approaches a drug-induced disease in humans. The toxicity of D-Galactosamine is mainly due to the collapse of uridine ponds that are linked with ribonucleic acid (RNA) and altering hepatocellular function (**Keppler & Jürgen 1974, 211-216**). This mechanism of toxicity increases cell membrane porousness leading to cell death. The cholestasis caused by galactosamine may be from negative effects on bile ducts. Galactosamine decreases the bile flow and its gratified i.e. bile salts, cholic acid, and deoxycholic acid. Dose of D-Galactosamine: 400mg/kg. i.p. (**Binduja Visen Dayal Agarwal *et al.*1996, 232**).

Thioacetamide Induced Hepatotoxicity

Thioacetamide is a selective hepatotoxic within a short period after the administration of the drug. It experiences an extensive metabolism of acetamide and thioacetamide S-dioxide by the mixed-function oxidase system (**Chieli & Gino 1984, 41-52**). Acetamide does not have liver necrotizing properties while thioacetamide S-oxide is further metabolized to cytochrome P-450 mono-oxygenase to sulfene, thioacetamide S-dioxide. The thioacetamide S-dioxide is an extremely reactive metabolite that is further oxidized to thioacetamide S-dioxide, which covalently dilemmas to liver, and macromolecules and initiates liver injury. Chronic exposure to thioacetamide produced cirrhosis in rats (**Pande Singh Khilnani Khilnani *et al.*1996,132-136**). The mechanism of thioacetamide toxicity is due to the formation of thioacetamide S-oxide which is responsible for the amendment in cell permeability and the concentration of Ca++ increases intracellular nuclear volume and also obstructs mitochondrial activity which clues to cell death (**Kaplowitz 2007, 334-348**).

1.3.1 Risk Factor of Hepatotoxicity

Several conditions are responsible for the development of hepatotoxicity. Liver injury involves certain risk factors that can be genetic, non-genetic, or environmental (**Snijdewind Colette Mieke Jeannine *et al.*2012, 409-416**). Adverse effects of drugs or metabolites (like, antiretroviral drugs and alcohol) and certain health conditions such as age, sex, and disease (HIV or diabetes) are coupled with each other (**Nanashima Mawatari Tahara Higuchi *et al.* 2012, 253-259**). Some recent research on hepatic injury and various disease condition Show increased hepatotoxicity among HIV, Diabetic, or Tuberculosis patient (**Daly & Chris 2009, 400-411**), (**Chalasani & Einar 2010, 2246-2259**).

1.3.2 Genetic facto

Idiosyncratic drug-induced liver injury (DILI) significantly associated with certain genetic traits and genetic studies conducted till now abundantly have been hypothesis-driven only, which involved a candidate compound–candidate gene approach (**Kwon Shin Sang Kim *et al.*2012, 132-136**), (**Andrade Mercedes Eugenia M. Isabel 2009, 1467-1487**). According to Jaewoo-kwon et al genetic variations in the thioredoxin reductase 1 gene (TXNRD1) leads to the development of DILI (**Kwon Shin Sang Kim *et al.*2012, 132-136**). Variations in the activity of drug-metabolizing enzymes, (such as CYPS3A, CYP2C9, and CYP2C19) which are required for drug metabolism lead to the pathogenesis of idiosyncratic DILI. Polymorphism of bio-activated pathway through CYP450 enzymes, detoxification reactions, and excretion/transport reaction together with immunological factors (HLA class II antigen, cytokines) are major genetic factors that can affect hepatotoxicity (**Wilke**

Debbie Dan Watkins ***et al.*****2007, 904-916**), (**Belland and Chalasani 2009, 337-347**).

1.3.3 Non Genetic Factor

Environmental factors like age, gender, drug dose, alcohol abuse, and some disease conditions like HIV, and TB are also associated with hepatotoxicity. For specific medication, age is an important risk factor for hepatotoxicity such as the use of aspirin at a younger age increases the risk of liver injury (**Larrey 2002, 145-156**), (**Lucena Raúl Fernández Pachkoria** ***et al.*****2006, 850-856**). A large-scale study on age factors in US patients has been done, which shows between 25 and 34 age hepatotoxicity is 4.4 per 1000 patients as it increases vigorously to 20.83 per 1000 patients at the age of 50 or older (**Zimmerman1999, 4-10**).

Women and men have different susceptibilities for drug-induced hepatotoxicity. For example according to Hyman and Zimmermanin in 1978 women are more susceptible to drugs like isoniazid, nitrofurantoin, chlorpromazine, etc. whereas men are mostly affected by azathioprine-induced hepatotoxicity (**Ekstedt Lennart Ulrik Holmqvist 2007,135-141**). Another factor obesity (increased expression of CYP2E1-associated condition), also responsible for liver injury acute and chronic alcohol consumption associated hepatotoxicity has been reported in various experiments. Some disease conditions like HIV tuberculosis, and Hepatitis B and C associated disease always increase liver injury (**Paumgartner Ulrich 2002, 525-531**).

1.4 Treatment of Liver Disease

Treatment options for common liver diseases such as cirrhosis, fatty liver, and chronic hepatitis are problematic. The effectiveness of treatments such as interferon, colchicine, Penicillamine, and corticosteroids are inconsistent at best and the incidence of side –effects is profound. Too often the treatment is worse than the disease. Physicians and patients require effective therapeutic agents with low incidence of side effects. Plants potentially constitute such a group. Several hundred plants have been examined for use in a wide variety of liver disorders. The latter category of plants includes: *Silybum marianum* (milk thistle), *Picrorrhiza kurroa* (Kutkin), *Curcuma longa* (Turmeric), *Camellia sinensis* (Green tea), *Chelidonium maju* (greater celandine), *Glycyrrhiza glabra* (Liquorice), *Allium sativa* (Garlic), *Andrographis paniculata*, *Phyllanthus niruri*, and *Eclipta alba* are proven hepatoprotective medicinal herbs, which have shown genuine utility in liver disorders. These plants are used widely in hepatoprotective preparations and extensive studies have been done on them. There are several phytoconstituents from plants that have exhibited hepatoprotective activity. Recent progress in the study of such plants has resulted in the isolation of about 170 different phytoconstituents from plants belonging to about 55 families, which exhibit hepatoprotective activity (**Hagey Crombie Edgard Martin *et al.* 1993, 1911-1917**).

1.4.1 Allopathic Treatment

Ursodeoxycholic acid, UDCA (Ursodiol)

At present UDCA is the only allopathic compound approved by the US FDA for the treatment of primary bilirubin cirrhosis (PBC) or hepatoprotection. It is increasingly being used to treat all cholestatic conditions because it improves serum liver (**Güldütuna Guido Matthias Bhatti *et al.* 1993, 1736-1744**). UDCA is a polar bile acid from cholangiocytes and the concentration of hydrophobic bile acid decreases intracellular thus reducing the toxicity of the bile. UDCA is a dihydroxy bile acid that is normally present in human bile in a small concentration of about 3% of total bile acids (**Schuetz Stephen Kazuto Valerie *et al.* 2001, 39411-39418**).

Multiple Actions of UDCA are as follows:

- Defence of injured cholangiocytes against toxic effects of bile acids.
  Hydrophobic bile acids damage cell membranes and use cytotoxicity at concentrations that are present in bile **(Velsor Kovacevic Kovacevic Leitner *et al.*2004, 10-19)**. UDCA may also protect cholangiocytes by falling apical uptake and UDCA encouraging basolateral efflux of bile acids from cholangiocytes and the concentration of hydrophobic bile acid decreasing intracellular thus reducing toxicity.
- Inspiration of Depollution of Hydrophobic Bile Acids.
  It has been documented that UDCA stimulates steroid breakdown. UDCA activates PXR in rat hepatocytes and induces CYP3A4, which is a bile acid- acid-metabolizing enzyme **(Weber Meinrad Stampfl 2003, 105-136).**

- Protection Against Bile Acid-Induced Apoptosis.
  Apoptosis is an important aspect of cell death in cholestasis liver diseases **(Wilke Debbie Dan Watkins *et al.*2007, 904-916).** Glycochenodeoxycholic acid induces apoptosis by ligand-independent activation of the Fas receptor in rat hepatocytes. UDCA shrinks Fas ligand-induced apoptosis in rat hepatocytes. It protects rat hepatocytes against bile acid-induced apoptosis by preventing bile acid-induced, c Jun N- terminal Kinase-dependent CD95 (fas) trafficking to the plasma membrane **(Winslow & Kroll 1998, 2192-2199).**

Clinical use of UDCA

- Biliary cirrhosis
- Biliary disease secondary to cystic fibrosis
- Non-alcoholic steatohepatitis, idiopathic chronic hepatitis
- Autoimmune hepatitis.
- Primary sclerosing cholangitis.
- Alcoholic hepatitis.

Penicillamine

Penicillamine is a degradation product of penicillin but has no antimicrobial activity. It was first isolated in 1953 from the urine of a patient with liver disease who was receiving penicillin **(Pugliese Vito Enrico Patrizia *et al.* 2021, 648).**

Mechanism of action: Penicillamine chelates several metals including copper, lead, iron, and mercury, forming stable water-soluble complexes that are renally excreted. It also combines chemically with cystine to form a stable, soluble, readily excreted complex. Although it usually takes months to a year for hepatic copper levels to decrease, clinical improvement is often seen in Bedlington Terriers after only a few weeks suggesting the drug has other beneficial effects other than copper depletion **(Sears 2013, 1-13).** Penicillamine induces hepatic metallothionein, which may bind and sequester copper in a nontoxic form. It may also have antifibrotic effects as it inhibits lysyl oxidase, an enzyme necessary for collagen synthesis, and directly binds to collagen fibrils, preventing cross-linking into stable collagen fibers. However, its efficacy as an antifibrotic agent in humans is doubtful and it has not been even evaluated in veterinary medicine. Penicillamine may have immunomodulatory effects and has been demonstrated to reduce IgM rheumatoid factor in humans with rheumatoid arthritis **(McQuaid Lamand Mason 1992, 744-750).**

Clinical applications: Penicillamine is a monothiol chelating agent that is used in veterinary medicine in the treatment of copper storage hepatopathy (e.g., Bedlington Terriers), lead toxicity, and cystine-urolithiasis. It has also been used in the management of rheumatoid arthritis in humans. Wilson disease is treated by trientine or penicillamine **(Sears 2013, 1-13) (McQuaid Lamand Mason 1992, 744-750).**

Other drugs

Other medications used to treat liver diseases may include ribavirin, lamivudine, steroids, and antibiotics. Wilson's disease is treated by trientine or penicillamine. Besides these many other drugs like Alphamethyldopa, halothane, INH (isoniazid), rifampicin, pyrazinamide, allopurinol, chlorpromazine, methyltestosterone, erythromycin, glibenclamide are used in various liver disease **(Aggarwal & Bhatt 2018, 1-13).**

1.4.2 Herbal treatment

Indian Traditional Medicine like Ayurveda, Siddha, and Unani are predominantly based on the use of plant materials. Herbal drugs have gained importance and popularity in recent years because of their safety, efficacy, and cost-effectiveness. Several Indian medicinal plants have been extensively used in the Indian medicinal for the management of liver disorders. The use of natural remedies for the treatment of liver diseases has a long history and medicinal plants and their derivatives are still used all over the world in one form or the other for their purpose. Scientific evaluation of plants has often shown that active principles in these are responsible for therapeutic success **(Rane Jadhao Bakal 2016, 24-36).**

Classification

These are generally classified into three classes without any strict declination among them

- Anti-hepatotoxic agents. These generally antagonize the effects of any hepatotoxins causing hepatitis or any liver disease.

- Hepatotropic agents. These generally support or promote the healing process of the liver. In practice, these two activities cannot be easily distinguished from each other.
- Hepatoprotective agents. These generally prevent various types of liver affections prophylactically. In general, any hepatoprotective agent can act as an anti hepatotoxic agent but the vice versa is always not true.

One constituent with a therapeutically proven claim from its hepatoprotective properties is silymarin. Glycyrrhizin, catechin, Saikosaponins, Curcumin, Picrolive Iand II, Gomosin, Acetylbergenin, Kolaviron **(Kashaw Nema Agarwal 2011, 360-374).**

1.4.3 Marketed Herbal Formulation Used for Liver Disease

Some of the very common formulations with their compositions are listed below:

A) Liv-52
It is a non-toxic hepatoprotective substance from The Himalaya Drug Co, BangloreLiv. 52 can improve the subjective condition and clinical parameters in patients with liver damage, in particular in alcoholic liver damage. Composition are *Achille amillefolium, Capparis spinosa, Cassia occidentalis, Terminalia arjuna* **(Kashaw Nema Agarwal 2011, 360-374).**

B) Limarin (Capsules and Suspension):
It has a potent hepatoprotective and free radical scavenging (antioxidant) action. Limarin is developed from the active extract of the fruit of *Silybum marianum* or the milk thistle. It is a European herbal product.

C) Cirrhitin:
Cirrhitin is a natural medicine formulated specifically to treat cirrhosis of the liver and marketed by CCNOW.

D) Sriliv (Capsules):
Hepatoprotective, Herbal capsule for Loss of Appetite, Alcoholic Liver Damage, Hepatitis, and Jaundice.

Some other polyherbal preparations such as Livex, HD-03, Hepatomed, Live 100, and Hepatoguard with proven efficacy are also used in different types of liver disorders **(Kashaw Nema Agarwal 2011, 360-374), (Bedi Reddy Bijjem Kumar *et al.*2016, 6-21).**

1.4.4 Medicinal Plants Having Hepatoprotective Activity

Many of the medicinal plants used traditionally have been established for their hepatoprotective activity by various researchers. A list of those medicinal plants having hepatoprotective activity is compiled.

Table 1-1 List of some medicinal plants having hepatoprotective activity (Khatun Rahman Kabir Akter *et al.* 2013, 38-41), (Wu & Ihsan 1996, 387).

Sl No	Name of the plant	Family	Part used
1	*Acalypha racemosa*	Eurphorbiaceae	Leaves
2	*Actinidias deliciosa*	Actinnidiaceae	Roots
3	*Achilleamille folium*	Asteraceae	Whole plant
4	*Aloe barbadensis Mill*	Liliaceae	Dried aerial parts
5	*Annona squamosal*	Annonaceae	Leaves
6	*Anoectochilus formosanus*	Annonaceae	Leaves
7	*Apium graveolens*	Apiaceae	Seeds
8	*Arachniode sexilis*	Dryopteridaceae	Rhizomes
9	*Artemisia absinthium*	Asteraceae	Powdered aerial parts
10	*Argemone mexicana*	Papaveraceae	Latex
11	*Azadirachta indica*	Meliaceae	Leaf
12	*Bacopa monniera*	Plantaginaceae	Whole plant
13	*Boerhaavia diffusa*	Nyctaginaceae	Roots
14	*Bupleurum kaoi*	Umbelliiferae	Dried root
15	*Camellia nut*	Theaceae	Seeds and leaves
16	*Cassia occidentalis*	Caesalpiniceae	Leaves
17	*Cassia tora*	Caesalpiniaceae	Leaves
18	*Carum copticum*	Apiaceae	Seeds
19	*Cassia fistula*	Leguminosae	Seeds
20	*Capparis spinosa*	Capparidaceae	Root bark
21	*Cajanus cajan*	Fabaceace	Leaves
22	*Calatropis procera*	Apocynaceae	Flowers
23	*Chamomile capitula*	Asteraceae	Fresh mature capitula
24	*Cichorium intybus*	Asteraceae	Leaves

25	*Celrodendrum inerme*	Verbenaceae	Leaves
26	*Cochlosperump lanchoni*	Coclospermaceae	Rhizomes
27	*Cordia macleodii*	Boraginaceae	Leaves
28	*Cochlospermum vitifolium*	Coclospermaceae	Bark
29	*Croton oblongifolius*	Euphorbiaceae	Aerial parts
30	*Cuscutas chinesis*	Convolvulaceae	Seeds
31	*Decaplepis hamiltonii*	Asclepiadaceae	Roots
32	*Embelia ribs*	Myrsinaceae	Fruits
33	*Equisetum arvense*	Equisetaceae	Aerial parts
34	*Euphorbia fusiformis*	Euphorbiaceae	Tubers
35	*Fumaria indica*	Papaveraceae	Whole plant
36	*Fructus schisandrae*	Magnoliaceae	Dried fructus
37	*Ganoderma lucidum*	Polyporaceaes	Winter mushrooms
38	*Ginkgo biloba*	Ginkgoaceae	Dried extract
39	*Glycyrrhiza glabra Linn.*	Fabaceae	Root powder
40	*Gundeliatouren fortii*	Asteraceae	Fresh edible stalk
41	*Hibiscus esculentus Linn.*	Malvaceae	Roots
42	*Hoslundia opposite*	Lamiaceae	Stem
43	*Hygrophila auriculata*	Acanthaceae	Root
44	*Hypercium japonicum*	Clusiaceae	Whole plant
45	*Juncus subulatus*	Juncaceae	Powdered tubers
46	*Kalanchoe pinnata Pers.*	Crassulaceae	Leaves
47	*Kigelia africana*	Bignoniaceae	Leaves
48	*Lactuca indica*	Compositae	Aerial parts
49	*Laggera pterodonta*	Asteraceae	Whole herb
50	*Luffa echinata*	Cucurbitaceae	Fruits
51	*Momordica subangulata*	Cucurbitaceae	Leaf
52	*Mallotus japonicas*	Euphorbiaceae	Cortex
53	*Momordica dioica*	Cucurbitaceae	Leaves
54	*Naragamia alata*	Meliaceae	Whole plant
55	*Nelumbo nucifera Gaertn*	Nelumbonaceae	Leaves
56	*Ocimum sanctum*	Lamiaceae	Leaf
57	*Orthosiphon stamineus*	Lamiaceae	Leaves
58	*Plantago major L.*	Plantaginaceae	Seeds
59	*Picrorhiza rhizome*	Scrophulariaceae	Dried underground stem

60	*Piper longum*	Piperaceae	Fruits and roots powder
61	*Ricinus communis*	Euphorbiaceae	Leaves
62	*Rubia cordifolia Linn*	Ruboaceae	Roots
63	*Saururus chinensis*	Saururaceae	Whole plant
64	*Schouwia thebica*	Arecaceae	Aerial parts
65	*Silybum marianum*	Asteraceae	Leaves
66	*Tecomella undulate*	Bignoniaceae	Stem bark
67	*Trianthema portulacastrum*	Aizoaceae	Leaves
68	*Trichosanthes cucumerina*	Cucurbitaceae	Whole plant
69	*Vitis vinifera*	Vitaceae	Leaves
70	*Vicia calcarata*	Fabaceae	Aerial parts
71	*Xylopia phloiodora*	Annonaceae	Stem bark and leaves
72	*Woodfordia fruticosa Kurz*	Lythraceae	Flowers
73	*Zanthoxylum armatum*	Rutaceae	Bark

2

AIM AND OBJECTIVE

BIMAN BHUYAN AND JENTINOCHET AMRI

Liver cell injury is caused by various agents such as certain antibiotics, chemotherapeutic agents, carbon tetrachloride, thioacetamide, excessive alcohol consumption, viral or bacterial infections, etc. **(Talwani, Gilliam, and Charles 2011, 111-130).** Unfortunately, conventional or synthetic drugs used in the treatment of liver diseases are inadequate and sometimes can have serious side effects (**Andrade and Paul 2011, 1431-1446).** Therefore, many folk remedies of plant origin are to be tested for their potential hepatoprotective activities. Herbal drugs are more widely used than allopathic drugs as hepatoprotective because of their better cultural acceptability, better compatibility with the human body, and fewer side effects **(Ali, Khan, Kaneez, Ali, *et al.* 2018, 199-215).** The present study was aimed at the evaluation of pharmacognostic characters and phytochemical analysis for standardization and identification of plants and also to evaluate the extract for hepatoprotective activity.

Ardisia humilis Vahl. is used in the treatment of jaundice, diarrhea, rheumatic arthritis, rheumatism, skin sore, and vertigo by the folk healers of Assam in their traditional care practice **(Shankar, Lavekar, Deb, and Sharma 2012, 124-129).**

Selection of plant (*Ardisia humilis* Vahl):

- Documentation, by interview of the traditional Healer, Practitioner, Vaid Hakim, etc.
- Recording of the whole process, by audio-visual method.
- Field survey with the traditional healer.
- Documenting the habitat of the plant.
- Documenting the biological diversity of the concerned area.

- Documenting the population, and abundance of the plant in its natural region.
- A photograph of the entire plant and part of interest was taken.
- Documenting the information regarding the collection time.

This study aims to carry out a pharmacognostic study and evaluation of the hepatoprotective activity of the leaves of *Ardisia humilis* Vahl with special reference to its putative protective role in carbon tetrachloride-induced liver toxicity on Wister albino rats.

The brief objective of the study can be stated as under:

- Collection and Authentication of the plant *Ardisia humilis* Vahl
- Microscopy and Macroscopy of fresh as well as dried plants.
- To investigate the pharmacognostic parameters of the crude drug.
- Preparation of extracts of the dried leaves of the *Ardisia humilis* Vahl by using different solvents.
- Phytochemical screening of the different solvent extracts.
- Development of Thin Layer Chromatography to detect the major photochemical constituents
- In-vivo study of an extract of *Ardisia humilis* Vahl with special reference to its putative protective role in CCl_4-induced liver injury on Wistar albino rats.
- Evaluation of different biochemical parameters viz. SGOT, SGPT, Alkaline phosphate, bilirubin, and cholesterol will be evaluated. Histopathological studies will be carried out after completing the experiment.
- Histopathological study of liver tissue, isolated after completion of experiment protocol.

3

Plan of Work

Biman Bhuyan

The work is proposed to be carried out using the following systematic protocol:

- Selection and collection of the plant
- Identification and Authentication of the plant
- Literature review
- Study of physicochemical parameters of the leaf
    - Ash value
    - Acid insoluble ash
    - Water-soluble ash
    - Extractive value
    - Alcohol soluble extractive
    - Water soluble extractive
    - Loss on drying
- Study of pharmacognostic parameters of the leaf
    - Study of macroscopical characters such as odor, shape, size, color, taste, etc.
    - Microscopical study
    - Fresh microscopy
    - Powder microscopy
    - Quantitative microscopy
    - Powdered drug analysis
- Preparation of the leaf extract by using a successive solvent extraction method.
- Primary phytochemical screening of different solvent extracts.
- Detection of major phytoconstituents in the extracts by TLC method.
- Acute toxicity study

- Evaluation of hepatoprotective activity in CCl_4-induced Wistar rat model.
- In vivo evaluation
  - Investigation of SGPT, SGOT, ALP, serum cholesterol, total and direct bilirubin, and total protein levels in the blood samples collected from animal groups.
  - Histopathological study of isolated tissues.
- Statistical treatment of data.

4

LITERATURE REVIEW

BIMAN BHUYAN, JENTINOCHET AMRI AND PRAKASH RAJAK

Documentation of traditional practices can be said to be the most basic and reliable tool used in drug discovery from traditional medicinal practices. Though the process of documentation of traditional medicinal practices is often tedious and interpretation of epistemology is difficult, when the exercise is designed meticulously, it generates impeccable outcomes and removes associated ambiguity.

This chapter reviews certain important literature about different aspects of the proposed study.

(Naik Priyadarsini Satav Banavalikar *et. al.*2003, 97-104) have studied four aqueous extracts from as many medicinal plants as mentioned in Ayurveda viz., *Momardica charantia* Linn (AP1), *Glycyrrhiza glabra* (AP2), *Acacia catechu* (AP3), and *Terminalia chebula* (AP4) for their potential as antioxidants. The antioxidant activity of these extracts was tested by studying the inhibition of radiation-induced lipid peroxidation in rat liver microsomes at different doses in the range of 100 600 Gy as estimated by thiobarbituric acid reactive substances (TBARS). Of all these extracts, AP4 showed maximum inhibition in the TBARS formation and hence is considered the best antioxidant among these four extracts. The extracts were found to restore the antioxidant enzyme superoxide dismutase (SOD) from the radiation-induced damage. The antioxidant capacities were also evaluated in terms of ascorbate equivalents by different methods such as cyclic voltammetry, decay of ABTS(.-) radical by pulse radiolysis, and decrease in the absorbance of DPPH radicals. The results were found to agree with the lipid peroxidation data and AP4 showed maximum value of ascorbate equivalents. Therefore AP4, with high antioxidant activity, was found to be the best among the four extracts.

(Roy Kamath Asad 2006, 305-311) has reported in his research work that the aqueous extract of *P. guajava* leaves showed good hepatoprotective activity when administered at doses 250 and 500 mg/kg orally and the effect observed was dose dependent. The lower dose did not show a hepatoprotective effect in chronic hepatic damage induced by CCl_4. The effect produced by the higher dose of aqueous extract of *P. guajava* leaves was similar to that produced by silymarin (100 mg/kg; p.o.), a well-known hepatoprotective agent.

(Nayak Marshall Isitor Adogwa 2011, 1-5) evaluated hypoglycemic and hepatoprotective properties of *Morinda citrifolia* in diabetes-induced rats. The fermented fruit juice of the *M. Citrifolia* (optical density = 1.25) was used for the study. Diabetes was induced by administering Streptozotocin (50 mg/kg body weight). Fasting blood glucose, body mass, liver tissue glycogen content, and the extent of liver degeneration were assessed. Diabetic experimental animals were treated with *M. citrifolia* juice (2 ml/kg, twice a day) and diabetic standard with reference hypoglycemic drug, glibenclamide orally for 20 days. Both the groups were found to exhibit a significant reduction in blood glucose levels of 150 mg/dl and 125 mg/dl, respectively, as compared to diabetics untreated with FBS = 360.0 mg/dl. On the 10th day of the experiment, diabetic experimental animals exhibited a decrease in body mass (10.2 g, 5.11%) which increased significantly by the 20th day (6 g, 3.0%). Histological study of liver tissue obtained from untreated diabetic animals revealed significant fatty degeneration as compared to the other three groups. The data of the study proved the hypoglycemic and hepatoprotective activity of *M. citrifolia*.

(Paramesha Chapeyil Venkatarangaiah Yelegara *et. al.*2011, 289-297) evaluated the hepatoprotective and *in vitro* antioxidant effect of methanolic extract and its isolated constituent, dehydroabietylamine, in *Carthamus tinctorious* L, var Annigeri-2-, an oil-yielding crop. The hepatoprotective effects were estimated for the parameters viz, total bilirubin, total protein, serum alanine amino transaminase (ALT), and serum aspartate aminotransferase (AST) and alkaline phosphatase (ALP) along with the pathological findings of hepatotoxicity. The *in vitro* antioxidant activity was evaluated by using free radical scavenging assays: DPPH, nitric oxide radical scavenging, hydroxyl radical, reducing power, ferrous ion chelating ability, and total antioxidant capacity. Both the methanolic extract (at 150 and 300 mg/kg bw) and dehydroabietylamine (at 50 mg/kg bw) showed significant liver protection against CCl_4-induced liver damage that was comparable with the standard drug, silymarin (100 mg/kg bw), in reducing the elevated serum enzyme markers. The liver sections of the animals treated with dehydroabietylamine elicit significant liver protection compared with the methanolic extract against CCl_4-induced liver damage. Further, both the methanolic extract and dehydroabietylamine exhibited a considerable and dose-dependent scavenging activity of DPPH, nitric oxide, and hydroxyl radical. Similarly, in the reducing power assay, the results were very persuasive. In addition, the Fe^{2+} chelating activity and the total antioxidant assay established the antioxidant property of the methanolic extract and its isolated constituent. Among the two experimental samples, dehydroabietylamine was found to be more effective for the said parameters.

(Eidi Pejman Maryam Jalal 2012, 495-507) have stated in his work that the administration of cinnamon extracts for 28 days significantly reduced the impact of CCl_4 toxicity on the serum markers of liver damage, aspartate aminotransferase, alanine aminotransferase, and alkaline phosphatase. The histopathological studies on rats also showed that cinnamon extract reduced the toxicity of CCl_4 and preserved the histoarchitecture of the liver tissue to near normal hence the cinnamon extract acts as a potent hepatoprotactive agent against CCl_4-induced hepatotoxicity in rats.

(Verma Masoodi Ahmed 2012, S1308-S1311) studied the antihepatotoxic activity of *Marrubium vul*gar L. through silico methods. The results stated that Vulgarin exhibited a significant antihepatotoxic activity by decreasing the elevated levels of serum enzymes like SGOT, SGPT, ALP, and total protein levels when compared to silymarin against CCl_4-induced toxicity in rats.

(Khatun Rahman Kabir Akter *et. al.* 2013, 38-41), stated that *Ardisia humilis* Vahl (Family- Myrsinaceae) has been traditionally used by the folklore medicinal practitioners of Bangladesh to treat cancer, heart disease, and liver poisoning.

(Magielse Arcoraci Breynaert Dooren *et. al.*2013, 250-256) had evaluated the hepatoprotective activity of aqueous decoction of *Desmodium adscendens* (Fabaceae) leaves and twigs against chemically-induced (D-pinitol) liver damage in rats. Enzyme levels of AST, ALT, and ALP, which are among the usual biomarkers for liver damage, and a significant decrease of AST and ALT was observed for the *Desmodium adscendens* decoction.

(Ramappa & Guruprasad 2013, 37-49) described in their review that the development of idiosyncratic hepatotoxicity is an intricate process involving both concurrent as well as sequential events determining the direction of the pathways, degree of liver injury, and its outcome. Several drug and host-related factors are associated with an increased risk of antituberculous drug-induced hepatotoxicity, although the majority of the studies are retrospective with varied case definitions and sample sizes. Investigations on genetic susceptibility to hepatotoxicity focused on the formation and accumulation of reactive metabolite as well as factors that contribute to cellular antioxidant defense mechanisms and the environment that can modulate the threshold for hepatocyte death secondary to oxidative stress.

(Selvam Venkatakrishnan Dhamodharan Murugesan *et. al.*2013, 305-308) conducted research to evaluate Hepatoprotective activity of methanolic extract of *Syzygium jambos* (Alston) (Linn.) leaves against Paracetamol-induced hepatic damage in Wistar albino rats was observed at two different doses, 100 and 200 mg/kg body weight. The healthy control, disease control, and standard drug *Silymarin*-treated groups were also maintained for the comparison. The liver marker enzymes SGOT, SGPT, ALKP, Serum Bilirubin, and other metabolic parameters like total cholesterol, and HDL-cholesterol were evaluated in all the experimental groups. The changes in liver function parameters were significant in comparison to the disease control group and the observed efficacy was comparable to standard drug. The efficacy of the extract was found to be dose-dependent. The histopathology study of the liver also supports the presence of hepatoprotective activity in *S. jambos* by showing improved cytoarchitecture of liver cells in the treated groups. The results obtained in this study indicate the necessity for further research on the isolation and characterization of functional molecules from the extract.

(Mallhi Qadir Khan Ali 2014, 60-66) had studied the ethnomedicinal use of *Morus nigra* (Family Moraceae) in the treatment of jaundice, diabetes, hypertension, cough, fever and cancer. The evaluation was conducted to determine the hepatoprotective activity of aqueous methanolic extract of leaves of *M. nigra*. Two doses of 250 mg/kg p.o and 500 mg/kg p.o showed that extract of *M. nigra* produced significant ($p<0.001$) reduction in liver enzymes (ALT, AST, ALP) and total bilirubin induced by paracetamol and the results are comparable to silymarin ($p<0.001$). Results were supported by histopathological investigations, phytochemical screening, and detection of active constituents by HPLC. The study showed that the aqueous methanolic extract of *M. nigra* possesses hepatoprotective activity that might be due to quercetin, luteolin, and isorhamnetin. It was concluded from this study that *M. nigra* has hepatoprotective activity against paracetamol-induced liver injury in mice.

(Saltos Blanca Luigi Nunziatina 2015, 1056-1064) conducted a bioassay-oriented approach that led to the isolation of 11 compounds, including three new natural flavonoids, (2S)-isookanin 7-O-α-L-arabinopyranoside, (2S)-isookanin 7-O-(2″-acetyl)-α-L-arabinopyranoside, and luteolin 7-O-β-D-glucopyranosyl-(1 → 6)-β-D-galactopyranoside, from *Bidens humilis* aerial parts. Their structures were determined via spectroscopic analyses including two-dimensional nuclear magnetic resonance. The antioxidant activity of all compounds was also tested by three different assays. The Relative Antioxidant Capacity Index (RACI) was applied therein, from the perspective of statistics, by integrating the antioxidant capacity data determined by the chemical methods.

(Basha Murthy Prakash Kirthi *et. al.*2016, 1107-1113) stated that *Ardisia* Solanaceae Roxb (Family- Myrsinaceae) has been traditionally used in cases of fever and pain whereas the leaf has hepatoprotective activity and the study reported the presence of tannins, alkaloids, flavonoids, saponin glycosides.

(Gulati Reshi Rai Ray 2018,1004) in their article have elaborately reviewed hepatotoxicity with special emphasis on the mechanistic pathways, experimental and preclinical evaluation procedure, and the relevant herbal protective strategies. Successful reference has been drawn regarding inflammation, immunomodulation, and oxidative stress are among the common biological mechanisms contributing to compromised liver function. A variety of drugs and chemicals were demonstrated to experimentally induce liver damage, which is assessed in the laboratory by physiological, biochemical, and pathological biomarkers.

(Hussain Khan Arshad Asif *et al.* 2019, 2285-2292) researched to evaluate the biological efficacy of *Cinnamomum zeylanicum* by pretreating Balb/c mice with cinnamon bark aqueous extract (200 mg/kg/day i.g.) 14 days before intragastrically administering a single toxic dose of acetaminophen (200 mg/kg). Blood samples were collected for analysis of biochemical and oxidative stress parameters and liver and kidney samples were collected for histopathological analysis. The results indicated that cinnamon aqueous extract exhibits a highly significant preventive potential by ameliorating APAP-induced elevated levels of serum alanine aminotransferase, aspartate aminotransferase, creatinine, urea, and macroscopic and histological alterations in liver and kidney. Moreover, a significant increase in total oxidant status and decrease in total antioxidant capacity accompanied by APAP exposure, were restored by cinnamon pretreatment. It was observed that prior administration of cinnamon prevented the toxic changes induced by acetaminophen as confirmed by histopathological examination, more possibly owing to its antioxidant potential. In conclusion, the pretreatment with cinnamon provides potential therapeutic applications in acute liver and kidney injury induced by APAP in an experimental animal model and it was demonstrated to have therapeutic potential in oxidative stress-associated diseases.

5

Plant Profile

Biman Bhuyan

Ardisia humilis Vahl. has been traditionally used by the folklore medicinal practitioners of Bangladesh to treat cancer, heart disease, and liver poisoning where cytotoxic, thrombolytic, and antioxidant medications are implicated. Besides, some other species of Ardisia were reported to have incriminated properties and chemical constituents **(Quattroachi, 2012, 365-366).**

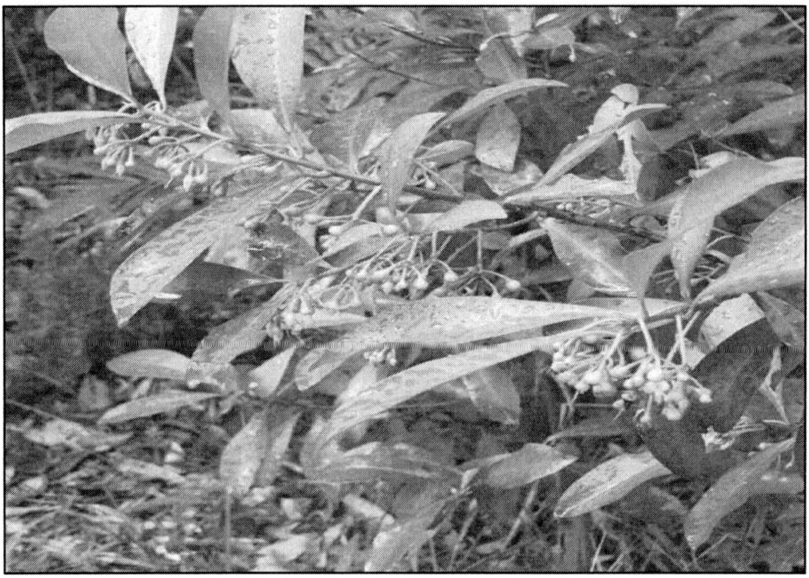

Fig. 5-1 Whole plant of *Ardisia humilis* Vahl

Scientific Name: *Ardisia humilis* Vahl.

Synonym: *Ardisia elliptica Rox.*

5.1 Vernacular Name (Randhawa and Mukhopadhyay, 2010, 132)

- Hindi name: Bisi
- Assamese name: Dhspon poita
- Marathi name: kadna,Katapenga,Bugadi,Dikna, nilbedsi
- Tamil name: Manipudbam,kozhikkottai,Narikandam
- Malayalam name: Kaka-njara
- Kannada name: Bodhina gida, Shudi,bode, Sore
- Bengali name: Banjam
- Oriya name: kuti
- Nepali name: Damaai phal

5.2 Botanical Description

Ardisia humilis Vahl. (Family: Primulaceae) is an evergreen shrub growing to 1-2m (rarely to 5m) tall. The leaves are broad ovate to elliptical, 15-18cm long and 5-7 cm broad, with a leathery texture and an acute apex. The flowers are reddish purple to pink, 5-6 mm in diameter; they are produced in corymbs in the mid-spring. The fruit is a red to dark purple drupe 6 mm diameter, containing a single seed, mature in the late autumn **(Oliver, 1994, 260-261).**

5.3 Taxonomical Description (Oliver, 1994, 260-261) (Wairt, 2006, 57-58)

Kingdom	Plantae
Order	Ericales
Family	Primulaceae
Genus	Ardisia
Species	A.*humilis*

5.4 Traditional Use

The plant *Ardisia humilis* Vahl was collected from the Madhuting region, Duliajan district of Assam. A verbal interview with Mr. Karuna Gogoi a traditional healer suggested that the paste of leaves of *Ardisia humilis* is used in the treatment of Jaundice and also in fever, diarrhoea, rheumatic arthritis, rheumatism, skin sore, and vertigo. Roots are used in fever, diarrhoea, and rheumatism and it has antibacterial activity. Juice extracted from the leaf and fruits of *Ardisia humilis* Vahl. can also be used as a stimulant and carminative.

6

MATERIALS AND METHODS

BIMAN BHUYAN, JENTINOCHET AMRI, AND PRAKASH RAJAK

6.1 Collection and Authentication of Plant Material

The *Ardisia humilis* Vahl. leaves were gathered in the month of September 2016 in the Madhuting region of the Duliajan district of Assam. The plant was identified and verified with reference number DU/PSC/HRB/B-01/2016 by Dr. S.K. Singh, Scientist-D, Botanical Survey of India (BSI), Shillong. The leaves were cleaned, dried for a month in the shade, and kept for use in the future.

6.2 Preparation of Leaf Powder of Ardisia *humilis* Vahl

Freshly gathered *Ardisia humilis* Vahl. leaves were air-dried for 25 to 30 days on a tray dryer at 35 ± 2 ºC. It was subsequently ground in a mechanical grinder to a fine powder with a mesh of 40 and stored in an airtight container for further investigation.

6.3 Pharmacognostic Evaluation

6.3.1 Macroscopic and Organoleptic Characters

A drug's evaluation entails verifying its identity, assessing its quality and purity, and identifying any adulterants, if any, if they are present. The aroma, taste, and texture of a crude drug are included in its macroscopy, along with its visual appearance to the unaided eye. Simple 10x magnification microscope was employed to observe specific structural attributes, including:

Size, shape, taste, odour, degree of regularity of the particles, colour, and external marking; surface appearance by reflected light, shining particles such as hairs, fibres, and calcium oxalate crystals; and size, shape, odour, and taste.

6.3.2 Microscopic characters

Thin transverse sections (TS) were cut by hand and dyed with safranin. The specimens were subsequently immersed in glycerine and examined under a microscope. **(Kokate 2006, 105-111), (Khandelwal 2004, 149-156).**

6.3.3 Powder Microscopy

Powder microscopy is one of the easiest and least expensive procedures for determining the identity of the source materials to begin with. It is useful for further pharmacological and therapeutic investigation as well as the standardisation of plant material. This aids in the observation and evaluation of cells in powdered form.

Procedure: Powdered plant material (leaves) was sieved through a 60-mesh sieve, cleared with chloral hydrate (clearing agent), stained with various staining reagents, mounted in glycerine, and then examined under a microscope. **(Wallis 2005,578-580).**

Photomicrographs: Wherever possible, microscopic descriptions of tissue are accompanied by micrographs; photos were obtained with a Canon digital camera. The scale bars show the magnification of the figures. Descriptive terms for anatomical features were included.

6.3.4 Quantitative Microscopy

- **Stomatal number:** It is the average number of stomata per square mm of the leaf's epidermis.
  Procedure: The leaf portions (middle section) were cleaned by boiling in potassium hydroxide solution and then peeled out of the upper and lower epidermis with forceps separately. It was mounted in glycerine water on the slide. A camera lucida and drawing board were set up to create a scale drawing. A stage micrometer was used to draw a 1mm square. The slide was placed on the stage, and the

epidermal cells and stomata were traced. The number of stomata in a 1 sq. mm area was counted. **(Khandelwal 2004, 149-156).**

- **Stomatal index:** The stomatal index is the ratio of the number of stomata to the total number of epidermal cells, with each stomata counting as one cell. The stomatal index can be determined using the following equation: **(Mukherjee 2002, 184-189).**

  $I = S/E+S\times 100$
  Where, I = Stomatal index
  S = No. of stomata per unit area
  E = No. of epidermal cells in the same unit area

  Procedure: The pieces of the leaf (middle part) were cleared by boiling with a potassium hydroxide solution and peeled out separately by means of forceps. It was kept on a slide and mounted in glycerine water. A camera lucida and drawing board were arranged for making the drawing to scale. A square of 1mm was drawn by means of a stage micrometre. The slide to be observed was placed on the stage, and the epidermal cells and stomata were traced. The number of stomata and the number of epidermal cells in each field were counted. The stomatal index was calculated using the above formula.
- **Vein-islet number:** A vein-islet is a small area of green tissue surrounded by veinlets. The vein-islet number is the average number of vein-islets per square millimeter of a leaf surface. It is determined by counting the number of vein islets in an area of 4 sq. mm. in the central part of the leaf between the midrib and the margin.
  Procedure: A piece of the leaf was cleared by boiling it in a chloral hydrate solution for about thirty minutes. A camera lucida and drawing board were arranged for making drawings to scale. A stage micrometre was placed on the microscope, and using a 16-mm objective, a line equivalent to 1 mm was drawn as seen through the microscope. The slide was placed with the cleared leaf (epidermis on the stage) and traced off the veins that are included within the square, completing the outlines of those islets that overlap two adjacent sides of the square. The number of vein islets was counted in square millimeters. The average number of vein islets was calculated from the four adjoining squares to get the values for one sq. mm. **(Raina 2003, 11–15), (WHO 1998).**

- **Vein termination number**: The vein termination number is defined as the veinlet termination per square millimeter of the leaf surface, midway between the midrib of the leaf and its margin. A vein termination is the ultimate free termination of a veinlet **(WHO 1998).**
  Procedure: A piece of the leaf was cleared by boiling it in a chloral hydrate solution for about thirty minutes. A camera lucida and drawing board were arranged for making drawings to scale. A stage micrometre was placed on the microscope, and using a 16-mm objective, a line equivalent to 1 mm was drawn as seen through the microscope. The slide was placed with the cleared leaf (epidermis on the stage) and traced off the veins that are included within the square, completing the outlines of those islets that overlap two adjacent sides of the square. The number of veinlet terminations present within the square was counted. The average number of veinlet terminations was calculated from the four adjoining squares to get the values for one sq. mm.

6.4 Physicochemical Parameters of Leaf Powder of *Ardisia humilis Vahl.*

6.4.1 Moisture Content (Loss on Drying)

To determine the amount of volatile matter (i.e., water drying off from the drug), the procedure given below was used. About 5g of accurately weighed drugs (accurately weighed to within 0.001) were taken in a tarred evaporating dish, dried at 105°C for 5 hours, and then reweighed. The percentage was calculated with reference to the initial weight **(Kokate 2006, 105-111), (Khandelwal 2004, 149-156).**

Formula:

$$\%\text{Moisture} = \frac{Fw - Pw}{W} \times 100$$

FW = Final constant weight of drug along with container
PW = Pre-weight of container
W = Total weight of drug taken

6.4.2 Determination of total ash

The determination of total ash is a method to measure the amount of the inorganic residual substance when the drug samples are ignited. Total ash determination involves detecting physiological ash (ash derived from plant tissue) and non-physiological ash (ash from extraneous matter, especially sand and soil adhering to the surface of the drug). For its detection, 2g of powdered material was placed in a suitable tarred container. The powdered drug was spread into an even layer and weighed accurately. The material was incinerated by gradually increasing the heat, not exceeding 450°C until free from carbon, cooled in a desiccator, weighed, and the percentage of ash calculated by taking into account the difference between the empty weight of the crucible and that of the crucible with total ash **(Govt. of India 2016, 111-139).**

Formula:

$$\%\text{Total ash} = \frac{Fw - Pw}{W} \times 100$$

6.4.3 Determination of acid insoluble ash

The ash obtained as per the above method was boiled for 5 minutes with 25 ml of dilute hydrochloric acid; the insoluble matter was collected over an ash-less filter paper, washed with hot water, and ignited to a constant weight. The percentage of acid-insoluble ash with reference to the air-dried ash was calculated.

Formula:

$$\%\text{Total ash} = \frac{Fw - Pw}{W} \text{ X } 100$$

Where, FW = Final weight of crucible with total ash
PW = Pre-weight of crucible
W = Total weight of powdered plant material

6.4.4 Determination of water-soluble ash

The total ash obtained was boiled for 5 minutes with 25 ml of water. The insoluble matter was collected on an ash-less filter paper, washed with hot water, and ignited to a constant weight at a low temperature. The weight of insoluble matter was subtracted from the weight of the ash. The difference in weights represents the water-soluble ash. The percentage of water-soluble ash with reference to the air-dried drug

6.4.5 Determination of loss on drying

2 g of the air-dried crude drug was accurately weighed in a weighing bottle and kept in a hot air oven maintained at 105°C for one hour or as specified. After cooling in desiccators, the loss in weight was recorded. This procedure was repeated until a constant weight was obtained.

Calculation

A = Bottle/Cover wt.
B = Sample + Bottle/Cover (Initial Wt.)
C = Sample Wt.
D = Sample + Bottle/Cover (Final Wt.)

$$\% \text{ LOD} = \frac{D-A}{C} \text{ X } 100$$

6.5 Extractive Values Determination

6.5.1 Determination of alcohol soluble extractive value

5 g of coarsely air-dried powdered drug was macerated with 100 ml of alcohol in a closed flask for 24 hours, shaken frequently for six hours, and allowed to stand for 18 hours. It was subjected to rapid filtration with precautions against loss of alcohol. 25 ml of the filtrate was evaporated to dryness in a tarred flat-bottomed shallow dish, dried at 105°C, and weighed. The percentage of alcohol-soluble extractive was calculated with reference to the air-dried drug **(Govt. of India 2016, 111-139).**

6.5.2 Determination of water soluble extractive value

5 g of coarsely air-dried powdered drug was macerated with 100 ml of chloroform water in a closed flask for 24 hours, shaking frequently for six hours, and allowed to stand for 18 hours. Then it was rapidly filtered, taking precautions against any loss of chloroform water. 25 ml of the filtrate was evaporated to dryness in a tarred flat-bottomed dish, dried at 105°C, and weighed. The percentage of water-soluble extractives was calculated with reference to air-dried drugs **(Govt. of India 2016, 111-139), (Gupta Sharma Ansari Lagarkha 2006, 249-251).**

6.6 Fluorescence Analysis

A small quantity of dried and finely powdered leaf sample was placed on a grease-free microscopic slide, and 1-2 drops of freshly prepared solution were added, mixed by gentle tilting the slide, and waited for 1-2 minutes. The slide was placed inside the UV viewer chamber and viewed under daylight and short (254 nm) and long (365 nm) ultraviolet radiation. The changes in colours observed by the application of different reagents to various radiations were recorded **(Gupta Sharma Ansari Lagarkha 2006, 249-251), (Kokoshi Kokoshi Slama 1958, 715-717).**

6.7 Phytochemical Analysis

Phytochemicals (from the Greek word phyto, meaning plant) are biologically active, naturally occurring chemical compounds found in plants that provide health benefits for humans beyond those attributed to macronutrients and micronutrients. They protect plants from disease and damage and contribute to the plant's colour, aroma, and flavour. In general, the plant chemicals that protect plant cells from environmental hazards such as pollution, stress, drought, UV exposure, and pathogenic attack are called phytochemicals. Recently, it has become clear that they have roles in the protection of human health when their dietary intake is significant. More than 4,000 phytochemicals have been catalogued and are classified by protective function, physical characteristics, and chemical characteristics, and about 150 phytochemicals have been studied in detail **(Owais Ahmad Khan Khan *et. al.*2006, 233-245), (Anonymous 2007, 235-340), (Meagher Thomson 1999, 105-114), (Wankhar Srinivasan Rajan Rathinasamy 2015, 17-21).**

6.8 Extraction Procedure

The shade-dried leaves were powdered, and 50g of powder was packed in a Soxhlet extractor for successive extraction with the following solvents:

1. Petroleum ether (60-80°C)
2. Chloroform
3. Ethyl acetate
4. Methanol

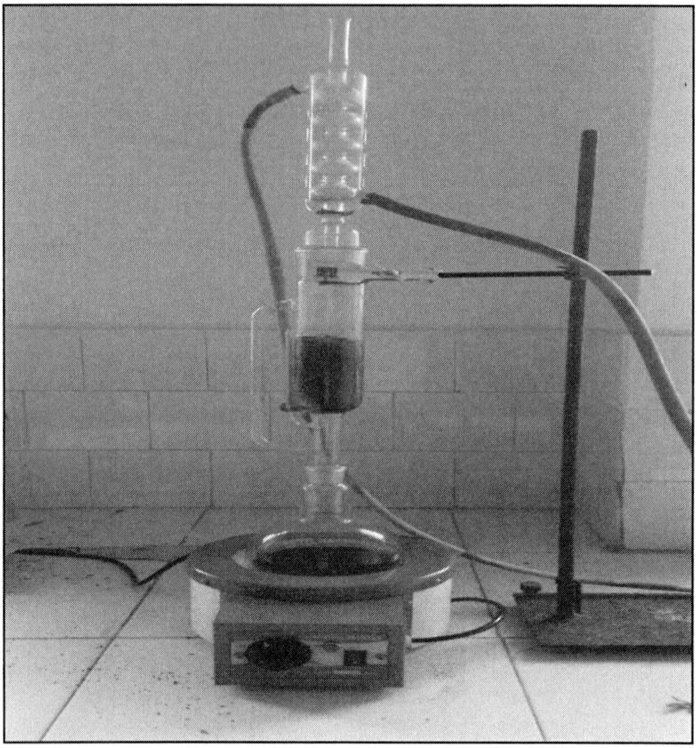

Fig 6-1 Extraction of powdered leaves

After extracting with petroleum ether for about 12 hours, the powdered material was first air dried and then oven dried below 40 °C. Then the material was extracted with chloroform for about 12 hours, and after completion, it was dried in a similar manner. The materials were further extracted with ethyl acetate and methanol in the same way. Each extract was concentrated by distilling off the solvent and evaporating to dryness in a petridish on a water bath **(Harbrone 2012, 1-36).**

6.9 Preliminary Phytochemical Tests

The different extracts obtained above were tested separately for the presence of various plant constituents, such as alkaloids, carbohydrates, glycosides, sterols, fats and oils, tannins, phenolic compounds, flavonoids, etc **(Evans2009, 133-147), (Colegate & Molyneux 2008, 12-65).**

1. Tests for Alkaloids:

A small portion of the extract was stirred separately with a few drops of dilute hydrochloric acid and filtered. The filtrate was then tested with the following reagents:

a. **Mayer's Reagent:** To 3 ml of filtrate, a few drops of Mayer's reagent (potassium mercuric iodide solution) were added and observed for the formation of a white or cream-coloured precipitate.
b. **Dragendorff's Reagent:** To 3 ml of filtrate, a few drops of Dragendorff's reagent (potassium bismuth iodide solution) were added and observed for the formation of an orange-brown precipitate.
c. **Hager's Reagent:** To 3 ml of filtrate, a few drops of Hager's reagent (a saturated aqueous solution of picric acid) were added and observed for the formation of a yellow precipitate.
d. **Wagner's Reagent:** To 3 ml of filtrate, a few drops of Wagner's reagent (iodine in potassium iodide) were added and observed for the formation of a red-brown precipitate.

2. Tests for Carbohydrates:

A small quantity of extract was dissolved in 5 ml of distilled water and filtered. The filtrate was then subjected to the following tests to detect the presence of carbohydrates:

a. **Molisch's Test (General Test):** To 3 ml of filtrate, a few drops of α-naphthol (20% in ethyl alcohol) were added. The mixture was shaken well. Then about 1 ml of concentrated sulphuric acid was added along the side of the test tube and observed for a reddish-violet-coloured ring at the junction of two layers.
b. **Tests for Reducing Sugars:**
   - **Benedict's test:** equal volumes of Benedict's reagent and test solution were mixed. The mixture was heated in a boiling water bath for 5 minutes and observed for the formation of characteristic coloured precipitates (green, yellow, or red, depending on the amount of reducing sugar present in the filtrate).
   - **Fehling's Reagent:** 1 ml of Fehling's solution A and 1 ml of Fehling's solution B were mixed and boiled for one minute. To

this, an equal volume of test solution was added, heated over a boiling water bath for 5–10 minutes, and observed for the formation of a brick-red precipitate.

c. **Tests for Pentose Sugars:** An equal amount of test solution and HCl were mixed, and a crystal of phloroglucinol was added and observed for the formation of a red colour.

d. **Test for Hexose Sugars:**

Cobalt-chloride test: 3 ml of test solution and 2 ml of cobalt chloride were mixed, boiled, and cooled. A few drops of NaOH solution were added. Solution observed for the formation of greenish blue (glucose), purple (fructose), or upper layer greenish blue and lower layer purple (mixture of glucose and fructose).

Tollen's phloroglucinol test for galactose: 5 ml of conc. HCl and 4 ml of 0.5% phloroglucinol were mixed, and 2 ml of test solution was added to it and heated. The formation of a yellow-to-red colour was observed.

e. **Test for Non-Reducing Polysaccharides (Starch):**

- **Iodine test:** 3 ml of the test solution and a few drops of dilute iodine solution were mixed and observed for the formation of a blue colour. The colour disappears on boiling and reappears on cooling.
- **Tannic acid test for starch:** With a 20% solution of tannic acid, the test solution was observed for precipitate.

3. Tests for Glycosides:

A small portion of the extract was hydrolyzed with dilute hydrochloric acid for one hour over a water bath, filtered, and then subjected to the following tests:

a. **Tests for anthraquinone glycosides:**

- **Borntrager's test for anthraquinone glycosides:** To 2 ml of filtrate, 3 ml of chloroform were added and shaken, and the chloroform layer was separated. A 10% ammonia solution was added to it and observed for the formation of a reddish-pink colour in the ammonia layer.
- **Modified Borntrager's test for C-glycosides:** To 5 ml of the extract, 5 ml of 5% $FeCl3$ and 5 ml of dilute HCl were added, heated for 5 min. on a boiling water bath, cooled, and benzene (or any organic solvent) was added. It was shaken well, the

organic layer was separated, and an equal volume of dilute ammonia was added and observed for the formation of a pinkish-red colour.

b. **Tests for cardiac glycosides:**
    - **Legal's test (Test for Cardenolide):** To the filtrate, 1 ml of pyridine and 1 ml of sodium nitroprusside solution were added and observed for the formation of a pink to red colour, which indicates the presence of glycoside.
    - **Liebermann's test (test for bufadenolide):** The extract was dissolved in 3 ml of acetic anhydride, and the mixture was heated and cooled. A few drops of concentrated sulfuric acid were then added and observed for the formation of a blue colour.
    - **Test for deoxysugars (Keller-Killiani Test):** To 2 ml of filtrate, a few drops of glacial acetic acid, one drop of 5% ferric chloride, and concentrated sulfuric acid were added. observed the formation of a reddish-brown colour at the junction of two liquid layers, and the upper layer appeared bluish-green in the presence of glycosides.
c. **Tests for Cyanogenetic Glycosides**
    Grignard reaction or sodium picrate test: A filter paper strip was first soaked in 10% picric acid, then in 10% sodium carbonate, and dried. The moistened powder drug was placed in a conical flask and corked; the above filter paper strip was placed on the slit in the cork. The filter paper was noted for its brick-red colour.
d. **Tests for saponin glycosides:**
    Foam test: The drug extract was shaken vigorously with water and observed for the formation of persistent foam.

4. Tests for steroids:

- **Liebermann-Burchard's Test:** The extract is dissolved in chloroform, and 1 to 2 ml of acetic anhydride is added along with a few drops of concentrated sulfuric acid from the side of the test tube. Observed for the formation of first red, then blue, and finally green colours.
- **Liebermann's test:** The extract was dissolved in 3 ml of acetic anhydride. Heated and cooled, then a few drops of concentrated sulfuric acid were added and observed for the formation of a blue colour.

- **Salkowski test:** To the extract, 2 ml of chloroform and 2 ml of concentrated sulfuric acid were added. Shaken well and observed for the formation of red colour in the chloroform layer and greenish-yellow fluorescence in the acid layer.

5. Tests for Fats and Oils:

- **Saponification test:** A few drops of 0.5 N alcoholic potassium hydroxide are added to a small quantity of the extract along with a drop of phenolphthalein. The mixture was heated in a water bath for 1–2 hours. The formation of soap or partial neutralisation of alkali indicated the presence of fixed oils and fats.
- **Spot test:** A small quantity of the extract was separately passed between two filter papers. The appearance of oil stains on paper indicated the presence of fixed oils.

6. Tests for Tannins and Phenolic Compounds:

To 3 ml of aqueous or alcoholic extract, a few drops of the following reagents are added:

- **5% Ferric Chloride Solution:** Deep blue or black colour
- **Lead acetate solution:** white precipitate
- **Acetic acid solution:** red colour solution
- **Potassium dichromate:** red precipitate
- **Dilute Iodine Solution:** Transient red colour
- **Dilute HNO3** to a reddish to yellowish colour.
- **Dilute potassium permanganate solution:**

7. Test for Proteins:

- **Biuret test:** 3 ml of test solution, 1 ml of 40% sodium hydroxide solution, and 2 drops of 1% $CuSO_4$ solution were added and observed for the formation of a pinkish or purple-violet colour.
- **Millon's test:** 1 ml of test solution was acidified with sulfuric acid added to Millon's reagent, boiled, and observed for the formation of a white precipitate. After warming, the precipitate turned brick red, or the precipitate dissolved, giving a red-coloured solution.
- **Test for proteins containing sulphur:** 5 ml of test solution was mixed with 2 ml of 40% NaOH and two drops of 10% lead acetate

solution. The solution was boiled and observed for the formation of a black or brownish-coloured solution due to PbS formation.

- **Xanthoprotein test:** To 1 ml of the extract, add 1 ml of concentrated nitric acid. A white precipitate was formed, and it was boiled and cooled. Then 20% sodium hydroxide, or ammonia, was added. Then it was observed that the formation of an orange colour was due to the presence of aromatic amino acids.
- **Precipitation test:** The test solution observed for the white colloidal precipitate was prepared with the following reagents:
  (i) 5% CuSO4 Solution
  (ii) 5% lead acetate

8. Tests for Amino Acids:

- **Ninhydrin Test (General Test):** To 3 ml of test solution, 3 drops of 5% Ninhydrin solution were added, heated in a boiling water bath for 10 minutes, and observed for the formation of a purple or bluish colour.
- **Test for Cystine:** To 3 ml of test solution, a few drops of 40% NaOH and 10% Lead Acetate solution were added, then boiled and observed for the formation of a black precipitate of Lead Sulphate.
- **Test for Tyrosine:** To 3 ml of test solution, 3 drops of Millon's reagent were added, heated, and observed for the formation of a dark red solution.

9. Test for gums:

The test solution was hydrolyzed using dilute HCl, and Benedict's or Fehling's test was performed and observed for the formation of red colour.

10. Tests for Mucilage:

A small quantity of the extract was added separately to 25 ml of absolute alcohol with constant stirring and filtered. The precipitate was dried in the air and examined for its swelling properties.

11. Tests for Flavonoids:

Shinoda test: a small quantity of the extract was taken in 5 ml of alcohol (95% ethanol), treated with a few drops of concentrated hydrochloric acid, and 0.5 g of magnesium turnings were added and observed for the formation of pink colour. To the small quantity of residue, lead acetate solution was added and observed for the formation of a yellow-coloured precipitate. The addition of an increasing amount of sodium hydroxide to the residue causes yellow coloration, which decolorizes after the addition of acid.

12. Test for Triterpenoids:

Noller's test: Two or three granules of tin metal were dissolved in 2 ml of thionyl chloride solution, and 1 ml of extract was added into the test tube and warmed; the formation of a pink colour indicates the presence of triterpenoids.

6.10 Thin layer chromatography (TLC)

6.10.1 Preparation of plates

Glass plates of 5 × 20 cm2 size were coated with silica gel G (E-mark and Co.) with the help of a spreader to a layer thickness of 0.25 mm. After spreading, the plates were first air-dried and then activated at 1100 °C for 30 min. After cooling, the plates were kept in desiccators until required for further use **(Evans2009, 133-147), (Colegate & Molyneux 2008, 12-65).**

6.10.2 Application of sample:

Usually, to get good spots, the concentration of the sample solution has to be a minimum of 2–5 μl of 1% solution of the test sample spotted using a capillary tube. The spots were placed equidistant from each other. The spotting area should not be immersed in the mobile phase. The spot should be just above the mobile phase in the chamber.

6.10.3 Mobile Phases:

Table 6-1 Solvent systems used for performing TLC of different extracts

Extract	Constituents	Solvent system
Petroleum ether	Fats and oils	Chloroform : Methanol : Acetic acid (25:10:1)
Chloroform	Flavanoids Phenolic Compounds Carbohydrates Phytosterol	Methanol: chloroform (15:1) Butanol : Acetic acid : Dist water (3:3:1) Toluene : Ethyl acetate : Formic acid (5:5:0.2) Toluene : Ethyl acetate (4.5:0.1)
Ethyl acetate	Fats and oils Flavanoids Phytosterol	Toluene : Ethyl acetate (9:1) Acetic acid : Formic acid : water (100:11:26)
Methanol	Flavanoids Phenols Tannin Glycosides Carbohydrates Phytosterol	Ethyl acetate : chloroform(4:6) Ethyl acetate : Carbon tetrachloride : Formic acid (2.1:1.1:1.1) Toluene : Acetone : Formic acid (6:6:1) Methanol : Ethyl acetate : water (6:3:1) Toluene : chloroform : Acetone (5:3.1:4.3)

6.10.4 Development of chromatogram

The extracts were spotted on the plates with the help of fine-bore capillaries, and a chromatogram was developed in a chromatographic chamber using different solvent systems at room temperature. In all cases, the solvent system was allowed to run at a distance of 10 mm from the point of application of the extract on the plates **(Evans 2009, 133–147).** The time required for the development varied from 15 to 20 minutes. After completion, the plates were removed from the chamber and allowed to dry in the air. These plates were observed under UV light at 254 nm (short wavelength) and at 365 nm (long wavelength) for the presence of spots, and the R_f values of the spots were calculated and recorded.

6.10.5. Determination of R_f (Retardation factor):

Retardation factor is the ratio of distance travelled by the solute to the distance travelled by solvent.

$$\text{Formula: } R_f = \frac{\text{Distance travelled by solute}}{\text{Distance travelled by solvent}}$$

The R_f value ranges from 0-1. However, ideal values are from 0.3-0.8.

6.11 Anti-oxidant activity

Living cells generate free radicals and other reactive oxygen species (ROS) as by-products of various physiological and biochemical processes. ROS are highly reactive molecules that include free radicals such as superoxide ions (O2-), hydroxyl radicals (OH-), nitric oxide radicals (NO), singlet molecular oxygen, peroxynitrite radicals, and hydrogen peroxide. ROS plays a major role in cell metabolism, including energy production, phagocytosis, and intracellular signalling in-vivo **(Ottolenghi 1959, 355-363).** However, these ROS produced by endogenous and exogenous sources can lead to a wide variety of pathological effects, such as DNA damage, carcinogenesis, and various degenerative disorders and neurodegenerative diseases. The most effective way to get rid of free radicals, which cause oxidative stress, is with the help of antioxidants. It has been reported earlier that antioxidants can prevent oxidative damage induced by reactive oxygen species as they can interfere with the oxidation process by inhibiting the initiation or propagation of oxidising chain reactions **(Shah Parmar Bhatt Chanda 2011, 188–194).** The human body uses an antioxidant defence system to neutralise reactive oxygen species. The system, which consists of enzymatic and non-enzymatic antioxidants and some antioxidant enzymes to protect against ROS, includes superoxide dismutase, catalase, glutathione peroxidase, and glutathione peroxidase. Non-enzymatic antioxidants include glutathione, tocopherol (Vitamin E), vitamin C, beta-carotene, and selenium. The antioxidants may be either natural or synthetic. Natural antioxidants such as ∞-tocopherol and ascorbic acid are widely used because they are regarded as safer and cause fewer adverse reactions. Natural antioxidants are considered safer and cause fewer adverse health effects than synthetic antioxidants.

6.11.1 Evaluation of antioxidant activity by DPPH radical scavenging method

Free radical scavenging activity of plant leaf extracts of *Ardisia humilis* Vahl was measured by 1, 1-diphenyl-2-picrylhydrazyl (DPPH). In brief, a 0.1 mM solution of DPPH in ethanol was prepared. This solution (1 ml) was added to 3 ml of different extracts in ethanol at different concentrations (5, 10, 15, 20, 25, 30 μg/ml). Here only those extracts are used that are solubilized in ethanol, and their various concentrations were prepared by the dilution method. The mixture was shaken vigorously and allowed to stand at room temperature for 30 minutes, then absorbance was measured at 517 nm by using a spectrophotometer (UV-VIS Shimadzu). The reference standard compound being used was ascorbic acid, and the experiment was done in triplicate. The IC50 value of the sample, which is the concentration of sample required to inhibit 50% of the DPPH free radical, was calculated using the log dose inhibition curve. A lower absorbance of the reaction mixture indicated higher free radical activity. The percent DPPH scavenging effect was calculated by using the following formula:

DPPH scavenging effect (%) or Percentage inhibition = **[Ao – A1/ Ao]× 100**

Where, Ao was the absorbance of control reaction and A1 was the absorbance in presence of test or standard sample.

6.11.2 Determination of total phenolic contents in the *Ardisia humilis* Vahl. extract

The phenolic compounds in the sample are oxidised using the Folin-Ciocalteu reagent. This reagent is a mixture of phosphotungstic and phosphomolybdic acids that are reduced by the oxidation of phenolic compounds in a mixture of tungsten and molybdenum oxides. The blue colour produced by the oxides has a maximum absorption at 760 nm and is proportional to the total phenolic concentration. The tannin content is calculated as the difference between the total and waste phenol contents.

Reagents:

1. Tannic acid (0.1 mg/mL, w/v): Dissolve 10 mg of tannic acid in 100 ml of distilled water.
2. Folin-Ciocalteu reagent (10%, v/v): Dilute 5 ml of Folin-Ciocalteu reagent with 45 mL of distilled water.
3. Sodium carbonate Na_2CO_3 (7.5%, w/v): Dissolve 7.5 g of Na_2CO_3 in 100 ml of distilled water. If necessary, solubilising the solution on a heating plate and magnetic stirrer.
4. Methanol (80%, v/v): Dilute 800 ml of methanol with 200 ml of distilled water.

6.11.3 Total flavonoid content determination

The total flavonoid content was determined with aluminium chloride ($AlCl_3$).

Quercetin was used as a standard. The plant extract (0.1 ml) was added to 0.3 ml of distilled water, followed by 0.03 ml of $NaNO_2$ (5%) and incubated for 5 min at 25 °C. Later, 0.03 ml of $AlCl_3$ (10%) was added, and after 5 min, the reaction mixture was treated with 0.2 ml (1 mM) NaOH. Finally, the reaction mixture was diluted to 1 ml with water, and the absorbance was measured at 510 nm. All tests were performed six times. The flavonoid content was calculated from a quercetin standard curve **(Saumya Mahaboob Basha 2011, 165-169).**

6.11.4 Nitric oxide scavenging assay

The activity was measured in 4 ml of the extract at different concentrations (1–50 μg/ml). 1 ml of sodium nitroprusside (SNP) solution (5 mM) was added and incubated for 2 hours at 27°C. An aliquot (2 ml) of the incubation solution was diluted with 1.2 ml of Griess reagent (1% sulphanilamide in 5% H_3PO_4 and 0.1% naphthylethylene diamine dihydrochloride). The absorbance of the chromophore was read immediately at 550nm and compared with the standard, and nitric oxide scavenging activity was calculated by the following formula **(Saumya Mahaboob Basha 2011, 165–169).**

Nitric oxide scavenging activity (%) = [Abs (control)–Abs (test)/Abs (control)] × 100

Where, Abs (control): Absorbance of control and
Abs (test): Absorbance of extract/standard.

6.11.5 Inhibition of Hydrogen peroxide radicals

The ability of the extract to scavenge hydrogen peroxide was determined. A solution of hydrogen peroxide (2 mmol/l) was prepared in phosphate buffer (pH 7.4). Extracts (1–10 g/ml) were added to a hydrogen peroxide solution (0.6 ml). The absorbance of hydrogen peroxide at 230 nm was determined after 10 min against a blank solution containing phosphate buffer without hydrogen peroxide and compared with ascorbic acid, the reference compound **(Ruch Cheng Klaunig 1989, 1003–1008).**

H_2O_2 activity (%) = [Abs (control)–Abs (test)/Abs (control)] × 100
Where, Abs (control): Absorbance of control and
Abs (test): Absorbance of extract/standard.

6.12 *In Vivo* Evaluation of Hepatoprotactive Activity

6.12.1 Selection of animals

Male albino rats of the Wistar strain weighing 100–200 g were used for the study. The animals were bought from Saha Enterprise, 386/2, Niluehal, Kolkata - 700051. All studies were performed in accordance with the guidance for the care and use of laboratory animals, as adopted and promulgated by the Institutional Animal Care Committee, CPCSEA, India. Regd. No.: 1828/PO/Bt/S/15/CPCSEA.

6.12.2 Maintenance of animals

The animal house was well ventilated, and animals were kept under conditions of 24 ± 2°C and relative humidity 44-56%, and 12 h light/12 h dark cycles each day for one week before and during the experiments. The animals were fed nutritional food and filtered water *ad libitum*. Animals described as fasting were deprived of food for ≥ 16 hours but allowed free access to water. The place where the experiments were conducted was kept very hygienic by being cleaned with an antiseptic solution.

6.12.3 Acclimatization of Animals:

Animals were kept for one week to acclimatise to laboratory conditions before starting the experiment; they were allowed free access to water and standard rat feed.

6.12.4 Preparation of leaf extract of *Ardisia humilis* Vahl

The dried powdered leaves were extracted with methanol by a hot continuous extraction process for 48 hours. The extract was concentrated by distilling off the solvent and then evaporated to dryness over the water bath. The dried extract was stored in a desiccator for further use.

6.12.5 Acute Toxicity Studies

Acute toxicity studies were performed as per Organisation for Economic Cooperation and Development (OECD) Guidelines 423. The institutional ethical committee of the Department of Pharmaceutical Sciences, Dibrugarh University, Dibrugarh, Assam, India, approved the experimental protocol (Approval No. IAEC/DU/129, dated December 29, 2016).

Healthy female Swiss albino mice (8–12 weeks old) were used for the acute oral toxicity study. The animals were randomly divided into 5 groups, each containing 3 mice, and marked on the tail to permit individual identification. The animals were housed in polypropylene cages for at least 7 days prior to dosing to allow for acclimatisation to the laboratory conditions. The temperature in the animal house was maintained at 22±3°C and the relative humidity was maintained at 30%, preferably not exceeding 70%. The lighting should be artificial, with the sequence being 12 hours of light and 12 hours of darkness. The animals were fed conventional laboratory diets with an unlimited supply of drinking water.

The test substance, i.e., methanolic extract, is administered in a single dose by gavage using a stomach tube or suitable intubation canula. The animals were fasted overnight prior to dosing (only water was provided). Following the period of fasting, based on the body weight of the animal, the amount of the dose was calculated, and the test substance, i.e., a methanolic extract sample, was administered orally at a dose of 5, 50, 300, 2000 mg/kg body weight. After the administration of the test substance, food was withheld for an additional 2 hours, and animals were observed individually at least once during the first 30 minutes, with special attention given during the first 4 hours and daily thereafter, for a total of 14 days. In **Table 6-2,** the total number of animals required is mentioned.

All the animals were observed at least twice daily for the purpose of recording any type of toxic effects caused by the test substance on the animal's health as per OECD Guidelines 423.

Table 6-2 Tabulated Break-Up of Total Animals Required (Acute Toxicity Study)

No. of Animals	Vehicle	Test Compounds to be Administered	Name of Group	Route of administration
3	0.3% CMC	--	Control	Oral
3	0.3% CMC	Extract 5mg/kg body wt.	Test dose 1	Oral
3	0.3% CMC	Extract 50mg/kg body wt.	Test dose 2	Oral
3	0.3% CMC	Extract 300mg/kg body wt.	Test dose 3	Oral

3	0.3% CMC	Extract 2000mg/kg body wt.	Test dose 4	Oral

6.13 Experimental Design for Hepatoprotactive Activity

The animals are to be divided randomly into six groups of six rats each. The hepatoprotective activity of the plant extracts was tested using the CCl_4 model (Fig. 6-2). Group I served as the control animal, which received a single daily dose of carboxymethyl cellulose (1 ml of 0.5% w/v, p.o. body weight). Group II received carbon tetrachloride (1 ml/kg body weight, i.p., a 1:1 v/v mixture of CCl_4 and olive oil) and 0.5% of CMC (1 ml/100 g). Group III received a dose of silymarin (200 mg/kg), while groups IV–VI received 400 mg/kg, 600 mg/kg, and 700 mg/kg of the extract of *Ardisia humilis* Vahl. in 0.5% w/v CMC (Table 6-3). The test doses were given orally daily, while carbon tetrachloride was given every 72 hours for 14 days. Animal blood was collected from the retro-orbtial vein and then sacrificed 1 hour after the last dose of the drug. The liver samples were dissected. The collected blood was allowed to clot, serum was separated at 2500 rpm for 15 minutes, and biochemical parameters were investigated **(Ruch Cheng Klaunig 1989, 1003-1008), (Sengottuvelu Srinivasan Rasalingam Jothive *et al. 2010*, 122-125).**

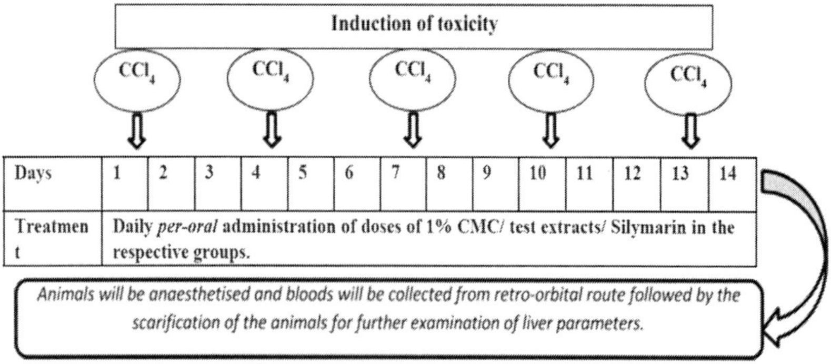

Fig 6-2 Study design of experimental animals

Table 6-3 Grouping of animals for experimentation

Group	No. of Animals	Induction of Hepatotoxicity	Treatment	Name of Group
I	6	Vehicle Control	0.5% CMC	Control
II	6	CCl_4(i.p)	0.5% CMC	Hepatic Control
III	6	CCl_4(i.p)	Silymarin (100mg/kg)	Reference Standard
IV	6	CCl_4(i.p)	Plant extract (300mg/kg)	Test 1
V	6	CCl_4(i.p)	Plant extract (500mg/kg)	Test 2
VI	6	CCl_4(i.p)	Plant extract (700mg/kg)	Test 3

CMC=Carboxymethylcellulose solution

6.14 Biochemical Parameters Investigation

6.14.1 Serum Glutamic Pyruvic Transaminase (SGPT)

SGPT is an enzyme that is normally present in liver and heart cells. SGPT is released into the blood when the liver and heart are damaged. The blood SGPT levels are thus elevated with liver damage (for example, from viral hepatitis) or with an insult to the heart (for example, from a heart attack). It is also called alanine aminotransferase.

Principle

ALT

Alanine aminotransferase (ALT) catalyses the transamination of L-alanine and α-ketoglutarate to form pyruvate and L-glutamate. In a subsequent reaction, lactate dehydrogenase (LD) reduces pyruvate to lactate with the simultaneous oxidation of nicotinamide adenine dinucleotide (NADH) to nicotinamide adenine dinucleotide (NAD). The rate of oxidation of NADH is measured kinetically by monitoring the decrease in absorbance at 340 nm. LD rapidly and completely reduces endogenous sample pyruvate during the initial incubation period so that it does not interfere with the assay **(Kaplan Amadeo Amin Ewa 1998, 752-757), (Doumas 1975, 1159-1166).**

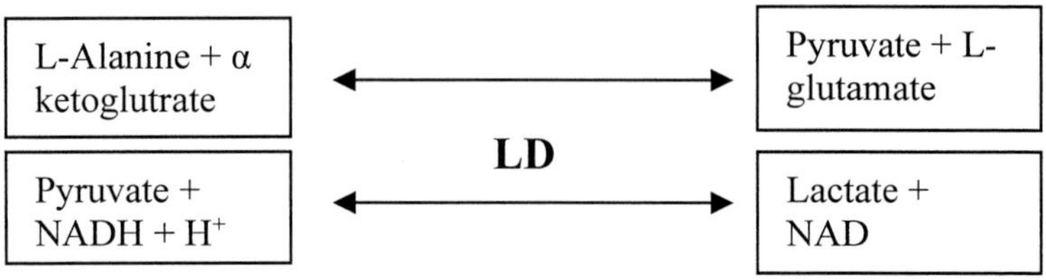

Reagent 1: Buffer
Reagent 2: Substrate

Working reagent preparation

Reagent 2 was added to reagent 1 in 1:4 ratio i.e. 1 ml of reagent 2+ 4 ml of reagent 1.

Procedure:

Pipette into tube marked	Test
Serum	100 μL
Working ALT reagent	1000 μL

1. Blank the analyser with purified water.
2. Absorbance was taken after 60 seconds and repeated taken after 30 seconds i.e. upto 120 seconds at 340 nm wavelength.
3. Mean absorbance was determined in change per minute.

Calculation

$$\text{AST activity(IU/L)} = \Delta\ \text{A/minute} \times \text{Kinetic factor}$$
$$\text{Kinetic factor (K)} = 1768$$

6.14.2 Serum Glutamate oxaloacetate Transaminase (SGOT)

SGOT is found in many tissues throughout the body, including the liver, heart, muscles, kidney, and brain. If any of these organs or tissues are affected by disease or injury, SGOT is released into the blood stream. Elevated levels of SGOT lead to myocardial infarction, cardiac operations, hepatitis, cirrhosis, acute renal diseases, and primary muscle disease.

Principle

Aspartate aminotransferase (AST) catalyses the transamination of L-aspartate and α-ketoglutarate to form L-glutamate and oxaloacetate. In a subsequent reaction, Malate Dehydrogenase reduces Oxaloacetate to Malate with simultaneous oxidation of Nicotinamide Adenine Dinucleotide [reduced] (NADH) to Nicotinamide Adenine Dinucleotide (NAD). The rate of oxidation of NADH is measured kinetically by monitoring the decrease in absorbance at 340 nm and is directly proportional to the AST activity in the sample. Lactate Dehydrogenase (LD) is added to the enzyme system to prevent endogenous pyruvate interference, which is normally present in the serum **(Kaplan Amadeo Amin Ewa 1998, 752-757), (Doumas 1975, 1159-1166).**

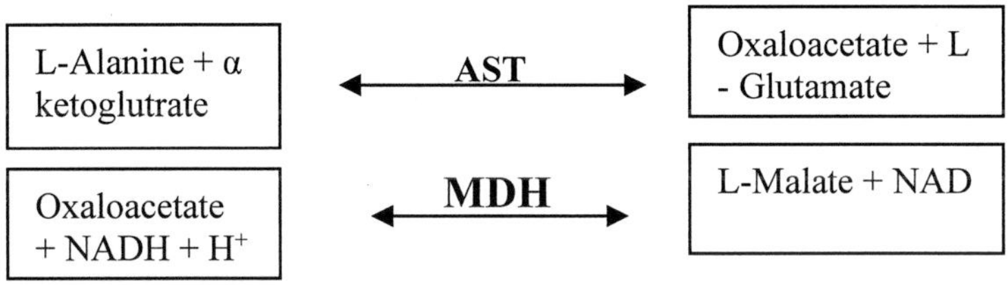

Reagents
Reagent 1- Buffer
Reagent 2- Substrate

Working reagent preparation

Reagent 2 was added to Reagent 1 in 1:4 ratio i.e. 1ml of Reagent 2 to 4ml of Reagent 1.

Procedure

Pipette into tube marked	Test
Serum	100 μL
Working AST reagent	1000 μL

1. Blank the analyser with purified water.
2. Absorbance was taken after 60 seconds and repeatedly taken for 30 seconds i.e. upto 120 seconds at 340 nm wavelength.
3. Mean absorbance was determined in change per minute.

Calculation

AST activity (IU/L) = Δ A/minute × Kinetic factor
Kinetic factor (K) = 1768

6.14.3 Total protein

A total protein test measures the total amount of protein in the blood. It also measures the amounts of two major groups of proteins in the blood, i.e., albumin and globulin. Albumin is made mainly in the liver. It helps to keep the blood from leaking out of blood vessels. This test is often done to diagnose nutritional problems, kidney disease, or liver disease.

Principle

Protein + CU^{++} ⟶ Blue violet coloured complex

The intensity of the coloured formed is directly proportional to the amount of total proteins present in the sample (**Ketcham Ashraf Madhavarao 2017, 117-123).**

Procedure

Pipette into clean dry test tubes labelled as-Blank (B), Standard (s), and Test (T)

Addition sequence	Blank	Standard	Test
Biuret Reagent	1000 µL	1000 µL	1000 µL
Total protein standard 6g/ml	—	10 µL	—
Serum	—	—	10 µL

All the solutions were mixed well and incubated at 37°C for 5 minutes. Then measure the absorbance of the standard and the test sample against the blank at 555nm (520–570) within 60 minutes.

6.14.4 Alkaline phosphatase (ALP)

Alkaline phosphatase is an enzyme found in the bloodstream. ALP helps breakdown proteins in the body and exists in different forms. It is mostly present in the liver, but some is also made in the bones, intestines, and kidneys. In pregnant women, ALP is made in the placenta. The ALP test can be helpful in identifying conditions such as hepatitis, cirrhosis, cholescystitis, and blockage of bile ducts.

Principle

Alkaline Phosphatase (ALP) catalyses the hydrolysis of p-nitro phenyl phosphate at pH 10.4, liberating p-nitro phenol and phosphate according to the following reaction:

$$\text{p-Nitrophenylphosphate} + H_2O \xrightarrow{\textbf{ALP}} \text{p-Nitrophenyl} + \text{Phosphate}$$

The rate of p-nitrophenol formation, measured photometrically, is proportional to the catalytic concentration of alkaline phosphatase present in the sample **(Raina 2003, 11-15), (WHO 1998), (Govt. of India 2016, 111-139), (Gupta Sharma Ansari Lagarkha 2006, 249-251).**

Reagent

R1Buffer:Diethanolamine(DEA)pH10.41mmol/L Magnesium chloride 0.5mmol/L
R 2 Substrate: p- Nitrophenylphosphate 10mmol/L

Reagent preparation

Working Reagent:

1 Volume of R_2 was mixed with 4 volumes of R_2

Procedure

Working reagent	1.0ml
Sample	20µL

1. Instrument was adjusted to zero with distilled water.
2. Mix and incubate for 1 min
3. Absorbance of the sample was taken at 1 min interval thereafter for 3 min.
4. Calculate the difference of absorbance and the average absorbance difference per minute (ΔA/ min) was calculated.

Calculation

$$\Delta A/\text{min} \times 2764 = \text{U/L of ALP}$$

6.14.5 Bilirubin (Total and Direct)

Bilirubin is an orange-yellow-pigment, a waste product primarily produced by the normal breakdown of heme. Heme is a component of hemaglobin, which is found in red blood cells. A bilirubin test is used to measure the level of bilirubin in the blood. It may be used to determine the cause of jaundice and help diagnose conditions such as liver diseases, hemolytic anaemia, and blockage of the bile ducts.

Bilirubin attached to sugar is called direct or conjugated bilirubin, and bilirubin without sugar is called indirect or unconjugated bilirubin. All the bilirubin in the blood together is called total bilirubin.

Principle:

Direct bilirubin reacts in an acid medium with the diazonium salt of sulphanilic acid to form a diazo compound (azobilirubin). The colour intensity is proportional to the concentration of direct bilirubin present in the sample.

Total bilirubin reacts in the presence of a quaternary ammonium salt in an acid medium with the diazonium salt sulphanilic acid to form a diazo compound (azobilirubin). The colour intensity is proportional to the concentration of total bilirubin present in the sample **(Tietz 1995, 10960-1106), (Bradbury Gordon Bancroft Stevens 1990, 119-42).**

Reagents

Reagent 1: Diazo-A
Reagent 2: Diazo-B
Reagent 3: Caffeine
Reagent 4: Methyl Red Standard

	Direct Bilirubin		**Total Bilirubin**	
Dispense	**Blank**	**Sample**	**Blank**	**Sample**
Diazo- A	50µl	50µl	50µl	50µl
Diazo- B	---	50µl	---	50µl
Caffeine	---		1000µL	1000µL
Distilled water	1000µL	1000µL	---	----
Sample	50µl	50µl	50µl	50µl

1. Mix and incubate at room temperature for 2 min.
2. Absorbance of the sample was taken against the distilled water blank.

Calculation

Concentration of bilirubin (Total and direct) in sample (mg/dl)

6.14.6 Cholesterol

Cholesterol is a fat-like substance that is found in all body cells. The liver makes all the cholesterol the body needs to form cell membranes and make certain hormones. The determination of serum cholesterol is one of the most important tools in the diagnosis and classification of lipemia. High blood cholesterol is one of the major risk factors for heart disease.

Principle

The cholesterol present in the sample originates in a coloured complex, according to the following reaction:

Cholesterol esters + H_2O Cholesterol + Fatty acids
Cholesterol + 4-Cholestenone + H_2O_2
$2H_2O_2$ + Phenol + 4-Aminophenazone Quinonimine +$4H_2O$

The intensity of the colour was proportional to the cholesterol concentration in the sample.

Procedure

	Blank	Standard	Sample
Reagent(ml)	1.0ml	1.0ml	1.0ml
Standard	---	10μL	---
Sample (μL)	---		10μL

1. Mix and incubate for 5 minutes at 37°C or 10minutes at room temperature (15-25°C).
2. The absorbance of the sample and standard were taken against the blank at 505nm.

Calculation

Cholesterol (mg/dl) = [Absorbance of the sample x 200 (standard concentration)/ Absorbance of standard]

6.15 Histopathological Study

6.15.1 Definition

It is a branch of pathology that deals with the study of disease in a tissue section.

6.15.2 Objective

1. To learn to understand the steps of the paraffin method of section preparation.
2. To prepare thin sections of an organ and learn something about its cellular structure.
3. To understand the importance of distinguishing "artifacts" from meaningful cell structures.

6.15.3 Paraffin method

All histological procedures can be divided into a similar series of steps. For the paraffin method, these steps are as follows:

i. Tissue resection
ii. Fixation
iii. Dehydration
iv. Infiltration and embedding in paraffin
v. Sectioning with a microtome
vi. Mounting on a microscope slides
vii. Clearing and staining
viii. Preparation of permanent mounts

The liver was removed and stored immediately in 10% buffered formalin. The tissue was fixed for at least 48 hours in buffered formalin 10%. The tissue was then cut and put in caste and this process was done next.

i. Improvement fixation: Formalin 10% - 0-3 hours
ii. Dehydration
    - 50% alcohol (10 minutes)
    - 70% alcohol (overnight)
    - 80% alcohol (30 minutes)
    - 90% and 95% (2 hours each, 2 changes)
    - Absolute alcohol (1 hour, 2 changes)

iii. Clearing with
   - Xylene – 1 hour
   - Xylene – 2 hour

iv. Impregnation: Liquid paraffin – 2.5 hours
   Liquid paraffin – 4 hours

6.15.4 Paraffin block preparation

After complete impregnation with paraffin, it is necessary to have solid blocks containing the tissues to facilitate proper sectioning of the material. The tissues in molten paraffin were poured into molds of suitable dimensions and the tissues were set properly within the paraffin. Orientation of tissues is important, which can be done according to the nature of the section necessary. To remove any air bubbles in the paraffin block the tip of the forceps were gently warmed, inserted, and passed around the specimen taking care to avoid any touch with the tissue. This is important as the presence of air bubbles in the block hinders proper sectioning. The molds were then gently immersed in cold water to cool the paraffin rapidly. This prevents the crystallization of paraffin. When the blocks became solid, they were removed from the water and detached from the mold with a scalpel. The tissues were then ready for sectioning.

Section cutting

The paraffin blocks were sectioned in a microtome to get serial sections, which come out in the form of a paraffin ribbon.

Materials

- Properly prepared tissues in paraffin block.
- Rotary microtome (Reichert – Jung), Hot plate.
- Microtome razor

Procedure

The excess paraffin at the sides of the block containing the tissues was trimmed to have a suitable size and fixed on a block holder of the microtome. The block holder was heated on a flame and pressed directly to the base of the block. The surface of the tissue was brought just below the knife edge by using coarse feed adjustment. The feed mechanism was adjusted to the desired setting of 5 μ. The microtome was operated and the section was cut. After having an 8`` ribbon, it was detached from the knife with the help of a scalpel and floated in a tray containing warm water. Small portions of this ribbon with serial sections were placed on clear glass slides and gently stretched using forceps or needles. Water on the slides was drained off and the slides were placed on a hot plate to allow the paraffin film to dry, set, and get attached to the glass slides.

Removal of paraffin wax

Paraffin being poorly permeable to stain, slides were dipped in xylene (to change each of 2-5 minutes) for complete removal of paraffin.

Removal of xylene

To remove xylene, the slides were placed in absolute alcohol for 3 minutes.

Dehydration

The slides were passed through descending grades of alcohol and finally washed in water for 3 minutes.

Staining

Double staining

To differentiate the nucleus and cytoplasm, the basic dye hematoxylin and the acid dye eosin were used.

Staining with hematoxylin

After washing in water, slides were treated with hematoxylin for 2-3 minutes

Development of colour

To develop the colour of hematoxylin, the slides were washed in tap water for 8- 10minutes

Staining with eosin

Since eosin was soluble in an alcohol medium but not in a water medium, the hematoxylin-stained slide was again passed through ascending alcohol grades with two final changes of 3 minutes each in absolute alcohol. The slides were placed from absolute alcohol to eosin solution and kept for one to one and a half minutes.

Treatment with absolute alcohol

Three changes each of 1 minute were given in absolute alcohol.

Clearing

Sections were treated with xylene 2-3 times for clearing.

Mounting

After treatment with xylene, a very small amount of DPX was placed over the section. Over this, a clean cover slip was pressed lightly to avoid the formation of bubbles. Slides were observed under an electrical light microscope and photographs were taken **(Lillie 1965, 942).**

7

RESULTS AND DISCUSSION

BIMAN BHUYAN, JENTINOCHET AMRI
AND PRAKASH RAJAK

7.1 Pharmacognostical evaluation

7.1.1 Macroscopic characters

The different macroscopic characters of *Ardisia humilis* Vahl. such as colour, odor, taste, shape are in Table 7-1.

Table 7-1 Macroscopic characters of the leaves of *Ardisia humilis* Vahl.

Sl. No.	Characteristics	Leaves
1	Colour of upper surface of leaf	Deep green in fresh form and greenish brown in dried form
2	Colour of lower surface of leaf	Green in fresh form and greenish yellow in dried form
3	Odour	Characteristic
4	Taste	Characteristic
5	Shape	Broad ovate to elliptical
6	Texture	Leathery texture
7	Size	15-18cm × 5-7cm
8	Margin	Entire margin
9	Apex	Acute

Discussion

The leaves are broadly ovate to elliptical with an entire margin. The colour of the upper surface of the leaf is deep green in fresh form and greenish yellow in dried form, and the lower surface of the leaf is green in fresh form and greenish yellow in dried form. It has a characteristic taste and a leathery texture with an acute apex.

7.1.2 Microscopic evaluation

7.1.2.1 Fresh microscopy

The different structures observed through microscopic evaluation of fresh leaves of *Ardisia humilis* Vahl. are given below in Fig. 7-1.

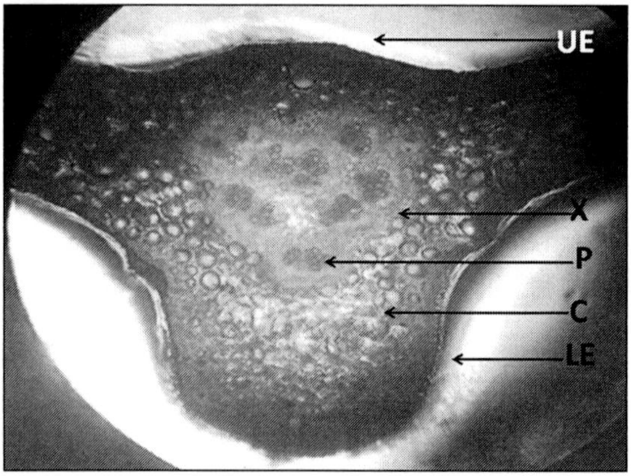

Fig 7-1 Transverse section of fresh Ardisia *humilis* Vahl. leaf
UE- Upper epidermis, X- Xylem, P- Phloem, C- Collenchyma, LE- Lower Epidermis

Discussion:

The transverse section of the microscopic leaf shows the lower and upper epidermis, with a tissue strengthened by cell walls known as collenchyma. Lignified xylem and phloem are also present.

7.1.2.2 Powder microscopy

The powdered characteristics of the leaf of *Ardisia humilis* Vahl. were studied and the results are given in Fig 7-2.

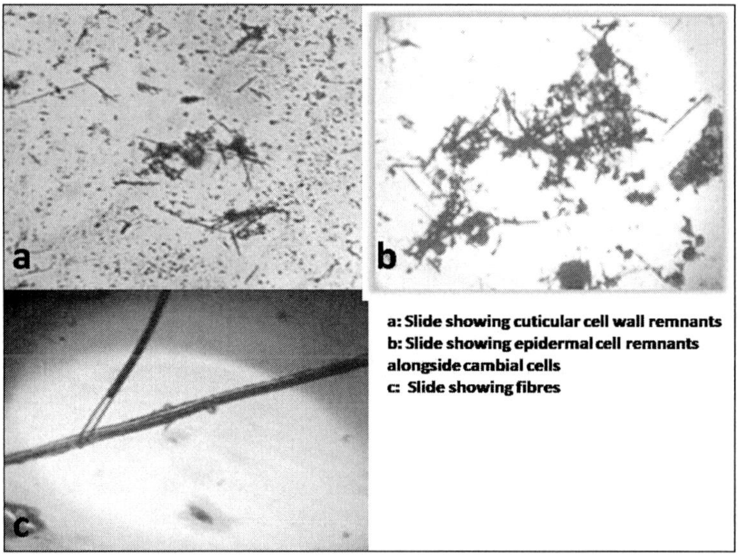

Fig 7-2 Powder microscopy of dried leaves powder of *Ardisia humilis* Vahl

Discussion:

The powder microscopy of *Ardisia humilis* Vahl leaf shows epidermal and cuticular cell wall remnants along with fibers.

7.1.2.3 Quantitative microscopy

In the quantitative microscopy, the stomatal number, stomatal index, vein-islets number and veinlet termination were determined and shown in Table 7-2.

Table 7-2 Quantitative microscopy of leaf of *Ardisia humilis* Vahl.

Sl. No.	Parameter	Value*
1	Stomatal number	65 ± 1.24
2	Stomatal index	20 ± 1.63
3	Vein-islet number	15 ± 0.82
4	Vein-termination number	18 ± 1.69

*Average of three readings ± standard deviation

Discussion:

Leaf constants are used as characteristics for the evaluation of plant drugs and their correct identification. A leaf constant such as stomatal number is affected by various factors like age, size of the leaf, etc. The stomatal index is not much affected by these factors. It is relatively constant. Hence, it is significant in the evaluation of leaf drugs.

The above-determined leaf constants of *Ardisia humilis* Vahl. are significant for the plant. It helps in the proper identification of plants. The value of the stomatal number was found to be 65 ± 1.24 per sq. mm, and the stomatal index value was 20 ± 1.63. The result of the vein-islet number was 15 ± 0.82, and the vein-islet termination number was 18 ± 1.69, which shows a significant value for *the Ardisia humilis* leaf.

7.1.3 Physicochemical evaluation

The values of physicochemical parameters of the dried leaf powder of *Ardisia humilis* Vahl. are given in Table 7-3.

Table 7-3 Physicochemical parameters of leaf powder of *Ardisia humilis* Vahl.

Sl. No.	Parameters		Results* (Mean ± SD)
1	AshValues	Total ash	11.40 ± 0.36
		Acid insoluble ash	6.45 ± 0.41
		Water soluble ash	9.14 ± 0.49

2	Extractive Values	Alcohol soluble extractive	6.45 ± 0.74
		Water soluble extractive	11.24 ± 0.65
3	Loss on drying		8.56 ± 0.52

*Average of three readings ± standard deviation

Discussion:

Physicochemical parameters such as ash value, acid-insoluble ash, water-soluble ash, alcohol-soluble extractive, and moisture content were recorded in the mean SD, which will help check the purity and quality of the drug (Table 7-3). Ashing involves the oxidation of the components of the product. A high ash value is indicative of contamination, substitution, or adulteration. The total ash usually contains carbonates, phosphates, and silicates, which include both physiological and non-physiological ash. Acid-insoluble ash usually indicates contamination with silicon materials like earth and sand. Water-soluble ash was studied for the estimation of the amount of inorganic elements.

The extractive value is also useful for the evaluation of crude drugs, which gives an idea about the nature of the chemical constituents present in a crude drug, and it is also useful for the estimation of specific constituents that are soluble in the particular solvent used for extraction.

Loss on drying is performed to measure the total change in weight of a material as a result of drying. Therefore, the LOD method measures both the water and volatile impurities in a sample under specified conditions. The objective of drying fresh materials is to fix their constituents, which are to check for enzymatic or hydrolytic reactions that might alter the chemical composition of the drug, and also to reduce their weight and bulk.

The results for total ash, acid-insoluble ash, and water-soluble ash were 11.40 ± 0.36, 6.45 ± 0.41, and 9.14 ± 0.49. Alcohol-soluble and water-soluble extractives show 6.45 ± 0.74 and 11.24 ± 0.65, respectively. Loss on drying shows results of 8.56 ± 0.52.

7.2 Fluorescence analysis

The results of the fluorescence study of the powdered leaves of *Ardisia humilis* Vahl. are given below in Table 7-4.

Table 7-4 Results of fluorescence analysis of leaf powder of *Ardisia humilis* Vahl.

Sl. No.	Particulars of treatment	Visible/ Day light	UV 365nm
1	Powder as such	Dark green	Dark green
2	Powder + 1N NaOH (Aq)	Brownish green	Green
3	Powder + 50% H_2SO_4	Green	Dark green
4	Powder + 1N HCl	Brown	Light green
5	Powder + Dragendroff's reagent	Greenish	Yellow
6	Powder + 50% HNO_3	Lemon yellow	Green
7	Powder + Ammonia	Pale brown	Brown
8	Powder + Iodine	Brown	Dark green
9	Powder + 5% $FeCl_3$	Dark green	Black
10	Powder + Acetic acid	Brown	Brown
11	Powder + 5% KOH	Greenish brown	Brown
12	Powder + Picric acid	Greenish yellow	Yellowish brown
13	Powder + H_2O	Dark green	Dark brown

Discussion:

In fluorescence analysis, the colour of the plant powder is mainly due to its chemical composition. They may appear at different wavelengths of light; it has been reported that specific colour patterns of various medicinal drugs are obtained at 365 nm and daylight. One of the important features of fluorescence is that UV light induces a fluorescent nature in many natural products where fluorescence is not seen in natural daylight. It will help to check the purity and quality of the drug. The powder drug exhibits different fluorescence characteristics due to the presence of different functional groups in its chemical constituents. In different proportions, the chemicals H_2SO_4, HCL, and HNO_3 in different proportions may change the configuration of the functional group present in the powdered drug, causing a colour change. The results of the fluorescence analysis of the powdered leaf are presented in Table 7-4.

7.3 Extraction of powdered leaves

The powdered leaves of *Ardisia humilis* Vahl. were successively extracted with petroleum ether, ethyl acetate, chloroform, and methanol. The percentage yield and extract observations are summarized in Table 7-5.

Table 7-5 Percentage yield of extraction of powdered leaves

Sl. No.	Extracts	Yield (% w/w)	Consistency	Color	Odour
1	Pet. Ether	3.25	Sticky-Solid	Dark Green	Characteristic
2	Ethyl Acetate	0.85	Sticky-Solid	Dark Green	Characteristic
3	Chloroform	1.75	Sticky-Solid	Dark Green	Characteristic
4	Methanol	11.23	Sticky-Solid	Dark Green	Characteristic

7.4 Phytochemical Screening

The different extracts were separately tested for the presence of various plant constituents such as alkaloids, flavonoids, glycosides, steroids, tannins, phenolic compounds, carbohydrates, saponins, triterpenoids, proteins, anthraquinones, and fatty acids. The results of the phytochemical tests are given below in Table 7-6.

Table 7-6 Results of Preliminary phytochemical screening

Sl. No.	Plant Constituents	Petroleum Ether Extract	Chloroform Extract	Ethyl Acetate Extract	Methanol Extract
1	Alkaloid	-	+	-	+
2	Amino acid	-	-	-	-
3	Carbohydrate	-	-	+	+
4	Fats and oils	+	+	-	-
5	Flavonoid	-	+	-	-
6	Glycoside	-	-	-	+
7	Lignin	-	-	-	-
8	Proteins	-	-	-	+
9	Phytosterol	+	+	+	-
10	Saponin	+	-	+	+
11	Tannin and Phenolic Compounds	-	-	+	+

Discussion:

In successive solvent extraction methods, four solvents are selected for the extraction of the leaf of *Ardisia humilis* Vahl. i.e., methanol, ethyl acetate, chloroform, and petroleum ether. Methanol has the highest yield percentage among all solvents. Preliminary phytochemical screening of the plant revealed the presence of different phytoconstituents.
A phytochemical investigation of various extracts showed the presence of various constituents. The petroleum ether and chloroform extracts revealed the presence of fatty acids and phytosterols. The ethyl acetate extract showed the presence of carbohydrates, saponins, phytosterols, tannins, and phenolic compounds. The methanolic extract revealed the presence of alkaloids, glycosides, carbohydrates, proteins, saponins, and tannins.

The preliminary phytochemical studies exhibited the presence of the maximum number of phytoconstituents in the methanolic extract.

7.5 Thin layer chromatography

Thin-layer chromatography was conducted on the different extracts using different mobile phases targeting different phytoconstituents. The results are compiled in Table 7-7.

Table 7-7 TLC profile of the leaf extracts of *Ardisia humilis* Vahl*000*.

Extract	Constituents	Solvent system	R_f value	Visualizing agents
Petroleum ether	Fats and oils	Chloroform: Methanol: Acetic acid (25:10:1)	0.58	Antimony chloride
Chloroform	Flavonoids	Methanol: chloroform (15:1)	0.57	Aluminium chloride
	Phenolic Compounds	Butanol : Acetic acid : Dist water (3:3:1)	0.73	33% ethanolic bismuth chloride solution
	Carbohydrates	Toluene : Ethyl acetate : Formic acid (5:5:0.2)	0.69	Benzidine
	Phytosterol	Toluene : Ethyl acetate (4.5:0.1)	0.61	
Ethyl acetate	Fats and oils	Toluene : Ethyl acetate (9:1)	0.86	Antimony chloride
	Flavanoids	Acetic acid : Formic acid : water (100:11:26)	0.35	Aluminium chloride
Methanol	Flavonoids	Ethyl acetate : Chloroform(4:6)	0.78	Aluminium chloride
	Phenols	Ethyl acetate : Carbon tetrachloride : Formic acid (2.1:1.1:1.1)	0.81	Chloramine trichloroacetic acid
	Glycosides	Toluene : Acetone : Formic acid (6:6:1)	0.75	Ethanolic bismuth chloride solution

	Carbohydrates	Methanol : Ethyl acetate : water (6:3:1)	0.87	
	Phytosterol	Toluene : chloroform : Acetone (5:3.1:4.3)	0.39	

Discussion:

TLC is produced to identify the individual substances present in a mixture and also for testing purity or separating mixtures. The R_f values indicate the position at which a substance is located in a chromatogram. It is appropriate to regard the R_f value as a guide for identification. Different mobile phases are selected, and iodine is used as a visualising agent for TLC determination. In the case of *Ardisia humilis* Vahl, methanolic and chloroform extracts showed the most prominent and maximum number of spots in that particular solvent system. All the solvent systems are efficient in the separation of phytoconstituents. The R_f values of different extracts in different solvent systems indicate the presence of different phytoconstituents.

7.6 Acute Toxicity Study

An acute oral toxicity study of methanolic extract was performed according to OECD Guideline 423 for testing chemicals. The main purpose of the acute toxicity study was to evaluate the toxicity profile of methanolic extract. A 14-day acute oral toxicity study was carried out on Swiss albino mice. The LD_{50} of the methanolic extract was not determined because the test substance did not produce any mortality up to a dose of 2000 mg/kg. No differences were found in the growth behaviour or body weight of animals between the control and test groups. The animals were observed twice a day up to 14 days, and observations are shown in Table 7-8.

Table 7-8 Observation Table for Acute Oral Toxicity Study

Sl. No.	Toxicity Sign	Observation
01	Convulsions	Not Occurred
02	Salivation	Not Occurred
03	Diarrhoea	Not Occurred
04	Lethargy	Not Occurred
05	Somatomotor Activity	Normal
06	Sleeping Disorder	Not Occurred
07	Behavioural Changes	Normal

7.7 In-Vitro Antioxidant activity

7.7.1 Inhibition of DPPH Scavenging Activity

In the DPPH radical scavenging assay, the extract exhibited concentration-dependent anti-radical activity by inhibiting DPPH radical. Ascorbic acid, which is a well-known antioxidant, showed a higher degree of free-radical scavenging activity than that of the plant extract at each concentration point. The IC_{50} value of the methanolic extract was 76.30μg/mL, while the IC_{50} value of the reference ascorbic acid was 38.5μg/mL. The extract was able to reduce the DPPH radical (visible as a deep purple colour) to a yellow-coloured diphynylpicrylhydrazine. This concludes that the plant might have active principles that can be used as antioxidants (Table 7–9).

Table 7-9 DPPH free radical scavenging activity of methanolic extract and standard.

Concentration (μg/ml)	Percentage Inhibition (Mean ± SD)	
	Ascorbic acid	MEAH*
10	32.56±0.32	21.61 ± 0.12
20	45.36±0.54	23.19 ± 0.36
40	52.35±0.36	30.75 ± 0.54
60	61.54±0.45	46.74 ±0.24
80	71.43±0.25	57.46 ± 0.35

*MEAH: Methanolic Extract of *Ardisia humilis* Vahl.

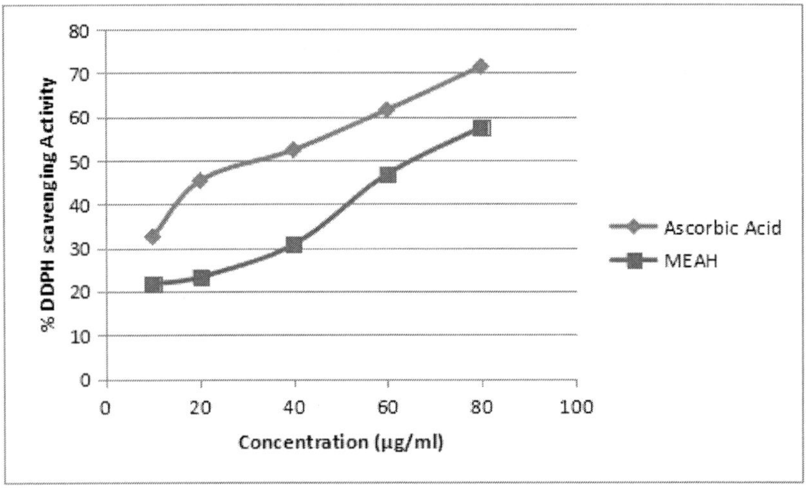

Fig.7-3 DPPH Scavenging activity of methanolic extract and standard

NO Scavenging Activity

The nitric oxide (NO) scavenging assay is based on the scavenging ability of the extracts as well as ascorbic acid, which is used as a standard. The scavenging of the NO generated from sodium nitroprusside in vitro indicates the possibility of preventing peroxynitrite formation in the cell *in vivo*. The scavenging of NO was found to increase in a dose-dependent manner (Fig. 7-4). The IC_{50} value of the crude extract was almost 100µg/mL, while the IC_{50} value for the reference ascorbic acid was less than 10µg/mL.

Table 7-10 Nitric oxide scavenging activity of methanolic extract and standard.

Concentration (µg/ml)	Percentage Inhibition (Mean±SD)		IC_{50}	
	Ascorbic Acid	MEAH	Ascorbic Acid	MEAH*
10	25.82±0.35	20.25±0.32	37.5	80
20	40.34 ±0.47	29.78±0.14		

40	53.72 ±0.35	36.31±0.34		
60	79.37 ±0.25	42.02±0.52		
80	83.8±0.29	50.3±0.63		

*MEAH: Methanolic Extract of *Ardisia humilis* Vahl

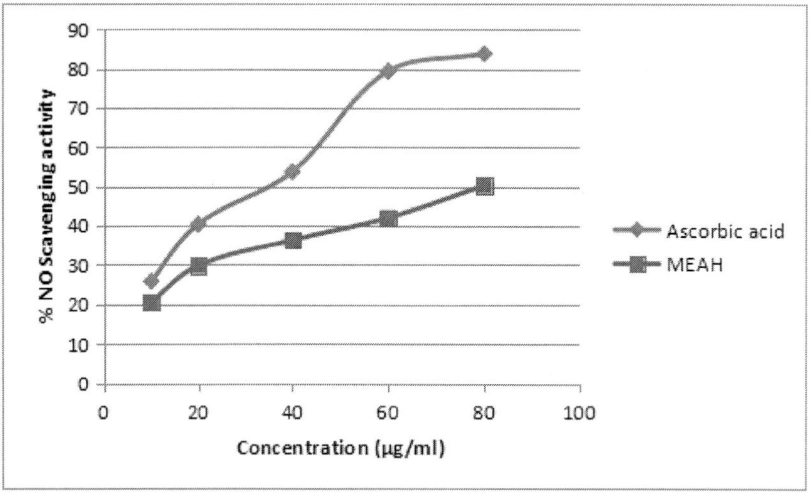

Fig.7-4 NO scavenging activity of methanolic extract and standard

Hydrogen Peroxide scavenging activity

The hydrogen peroxide (H_2O_2) scavenging assay is based on the scavenging ability of the extracts as well as ascorbic acid, which is used as a standard. The scavenging of H_2O_2 was found to increase in a dose-dependent manner (Fig. 7–5). The IC_{50} value of the crude extract was above 100 μg/mL, while the IC_{50} value for the reference ascorbic acid was about 60μg/mL. Based on these, we can determine the scavenging activity of *Ardisia humilis* Vahl. may have H_2O_2 radical scavenging activity.

Table 7-11 Hydrogen Peroxide scavenging activity of methanolic extract and standard.

Concentration (μg/ml)	Percentage Inhibition (Mean±SD)		IC_{50}	
	Ascorbic Acid	MEAH*	Ascorbic Acid	MEAH*
10	42.17±0.15	31.21±0.36		
20	45.14±0.36	36.52±0.45		
40	51.45±0.42	45.51±0.36	37.2	81.5
60	60.43±0.36	49.85±0.27		
80	65.53±0.24	56.32±0.34		

*MEAH: Methanolic Extract of *Ardisia humilis* Vahl

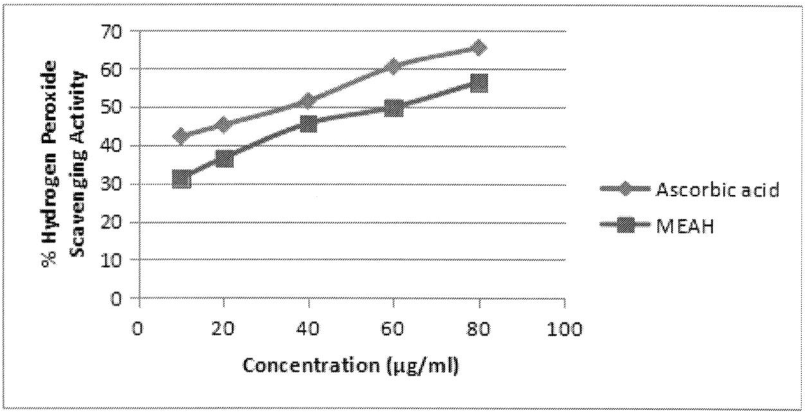

Fig 7-5 Hydrogen peroxide scavenging activity of methanolic extract

Discussion:

The in vitro antioxidant study was carried out by the DPPH free radical scavenging method, the nitric oxide scavenging method, and the hydroxy radical scavenging method. The IC_{50} value was determined for each method for standard (ascorbic acid) and Methanolic extracts of *Ardisia humilis* Vahl plant. The current study showed that the Methanolic extract contains a significant amount of antioxidants.

7.8 In-Vivo Evaluation of Hepatoprotactive Activity

7.8.1 Body weight and temperature

During the experiment the deviation of body weight and body temperature were measured and noted in Table 7-12 and 7-13.

Table 7-12 Body weight (in g) variation of the animals during experiments

Group	Body weight (g) (mean±SD) 0th day	Body weight (g) (mean±SD) 5^{th}day	Body weight (g) (mean±SD) 10th day	Body weight (g) (mean±SD) 14th day
G-I Vehicle Control	89.75 ± 8.09	90.13 ± 8.08	90.71 ± 8.05	91.55 ± 7.92
G-II Hepatic Control	98.33 ± 4.83	99.00 ± 4.82	100.11 ± 4.95	101.01 ±4.89
G-III Standard Drug	88.71 ± 12.92	89.23 ± 12.91	90.11 ± 12.88	91.25 ± 12.57
G-IV Test 1 (300mg/kg)	66.2± 7.311	66.91± 7.43	69.5± 9.61	71.15± 9.872
G-V Test 2 (500mg/kg)	115.95± 9.830	116.81± 9.92	117.56± 10.01	118.28± 10.06
G-VI Test 3 (700mg/kg)	88.66± 16.07	89.48± 16.15	90.266± 16.26	91.13± 16.31

Table 7-13 Temperature variation of the animals during experiment

Group	Temp. (^{0}F) (mean±SD) 0th day	Temp. (^{0}F) (mean±SD) 5^{th}day	Temp. (^{0}F) (mean±SD) 10th day	Temp. (^{0}F) (mean±SD) 14th day
G-I Vehicle Control	98.44 ± 0.157	98.43 ± 0.172	98.04 ± 0.499	97.71 ± 0.519
G-II Hepatic Control	98.14 ± 0.642	97.74 ± 0.642	98.25 ± 0.862	97.52 ± 0.443
G-III Standard Drug	97.47 ± 0.927	97.56 ± 0.926	98.15 ± 0.562	97.22 ± 0.793

G-IV Test 1 (300mg/kg)	98.02 ± 0.33	96.15 ± 0.65	98.29 ± 0.47	97.25 ± 0.31
G-V Test 2 (500mg/kg)	97.26 ± 0.26	98.12 ± 0.22	98.26 ± 0.82	96.56 ± 0.34
G-VI Test 3 (700mg/kg)	97.76 ± 0.64	97.35 ± 0.82	97.29 ± 0.42	98.45 ± 0.24

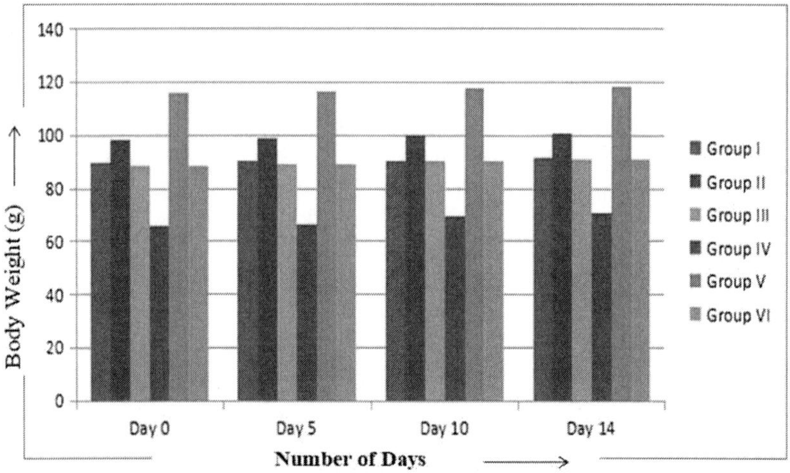

Fig 7-6 Graphical presentation of body weight variation of the animals

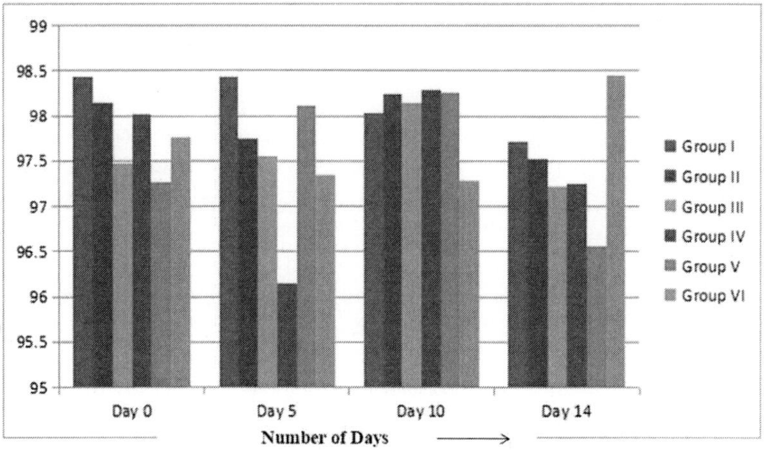

Fig 7-7 Graphical presentation of temperature variation of the animals

7.8.2 Bio-chemical parameters

The effect of different doses of methanolic extracts of the leaves on the SGPT, SGOT, ALP, cholesterol, total and direct bilirubin, and total protein levels was investigated in the carbon tetrachloride-induced albino rats using Silymarin as a standard drug. The results are summarized in Tables 7-14 & 7-15

Table 7-14 Effects of methanolic extract of *Ardisia humilis* Vahl. on SGOT, SGPT, ALP and cholesterol levels in experimental animals

Group	SGOT(U/L) (mean±SD)	SGPT(U/L) (mean±SD)	LP(U/L) (mean±SD)	Cholesterol (mmol/L) (mean±SD)
G-I Vehicle Control	55.03±0.872 **	48.311±0.52 0**	102.53±0.62 7**	182.48±0.52 2**
G-II Hepatic Control	107.86±0.88 1**	95.57± 0.572**	167.10±0.74 9**	145.36±0.52 7**
G-III Standard Drug	62.03±0.782 9	56.55±0.718	127.58±0.49 7	158.90±0.43 5

G-IV Test 1 (300mg/kg)	88.25±0.316**	84.97±0.206**	150.28±0.346**	144.44±0.638**
G-V Test 2 (500mg/kg)	78.81±0.366**	72.77±0.353**	141.22±0.810**	164.37±0.510**
G-VI Test 3 (700mg/kg)	83.12±0.317**	78.344±0.332**	146.14±0.192**	165.02±0.355**

** Values are significant with comparison to standard control (p<0.01), using Dunnett compare test Vs standard control.

Table 7-15 Effects of methanolic extract of *Ardisia humilis* Vahl. on direct bilirubin and total protein levels in experimental animals

Group	Total Bilirubin (mg/dl) (mean±SD)	Total protein (mg/dl) (mean±SD)
G-I Vehicle Control	0.63 ± 0.021**	8.15 ± 0.012**
G-II Hepatic Control	1.86 ± 0.006**	4.26 ± 0.015**
G-III Standard Drug	0.724 ± 0.005	7.37 ± 0.156
G-IV Test 1 (300mg/kg)	1.180 ± 0.003**	5.89 ± 0.028**
G-V Test 2 (500mg/kg)	0.822 ± 0.005**	6.86 ± 0.060**
G-VI Test 3 (700mg/kg)	0.876 ± 0.002**	6.23 ± 6.120**

** Values are significant with comparison to standard control (p<0.01), using Dunnett compare test Vs standard control.

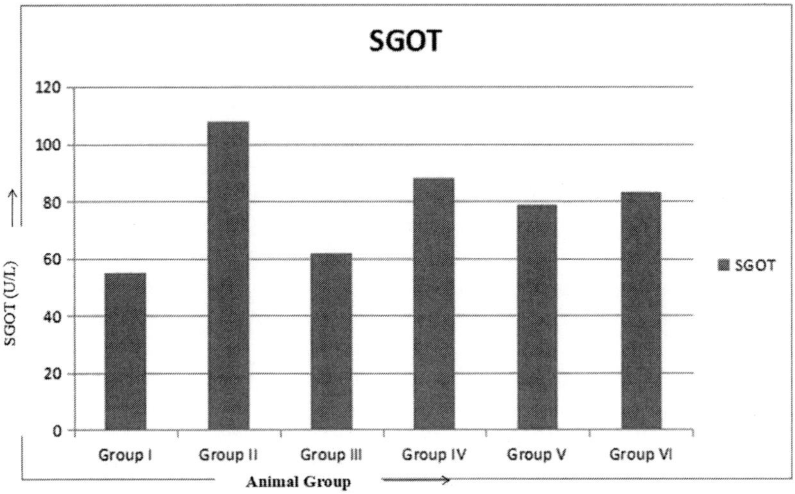

Fig 7-8 Graphical presentation of SGOT

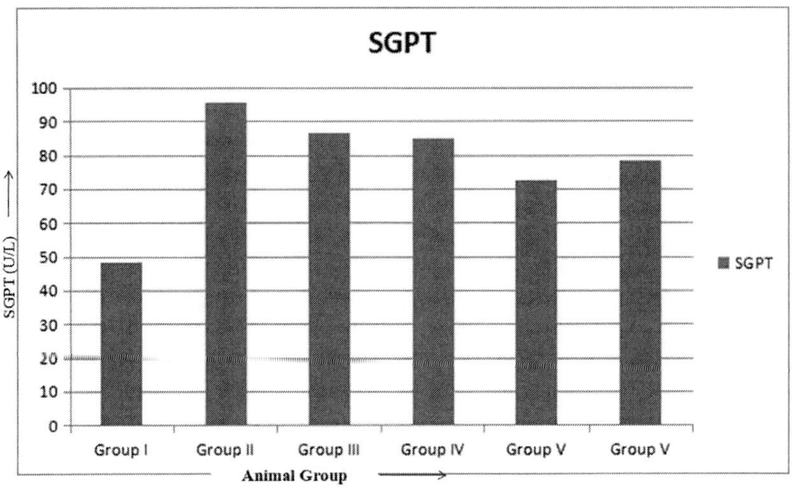

Fig 7-9 Graphical presentation of SGPT

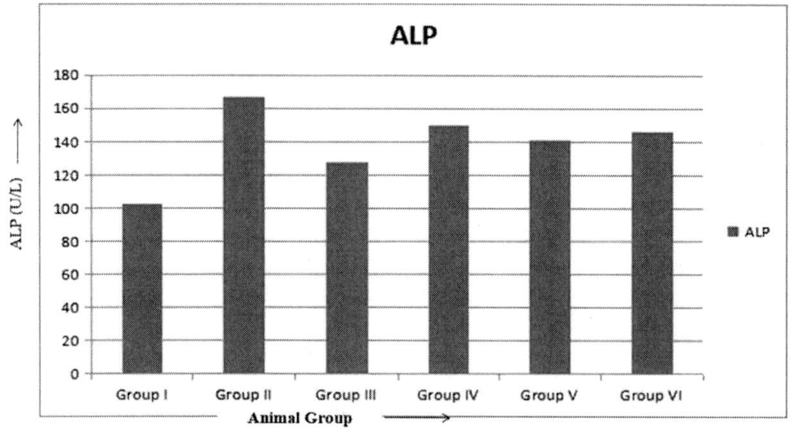

Fig 7-10 Graphical presentation of ALP

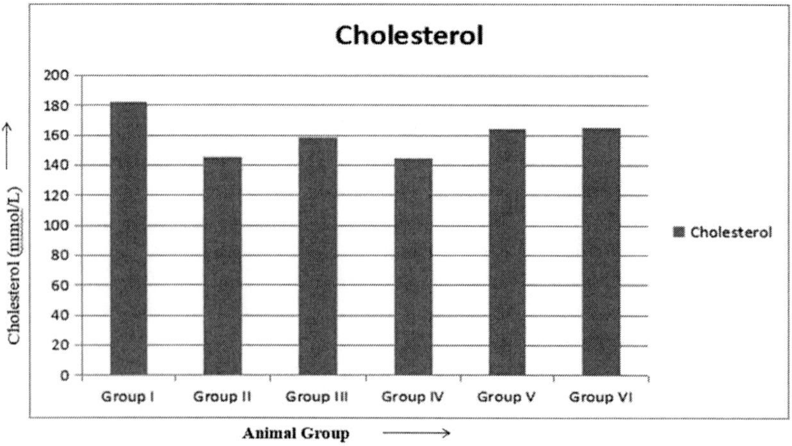

Fig 7-11 Graphical presentation of cholesterol

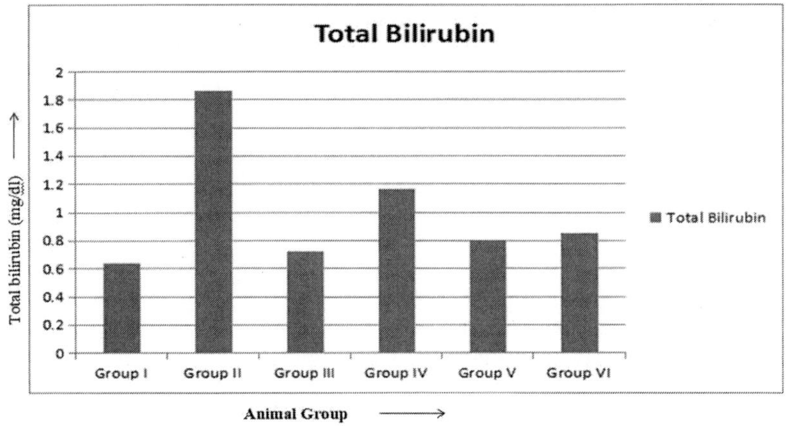

Fig 7-12 Graphical presentation of total bilirubin

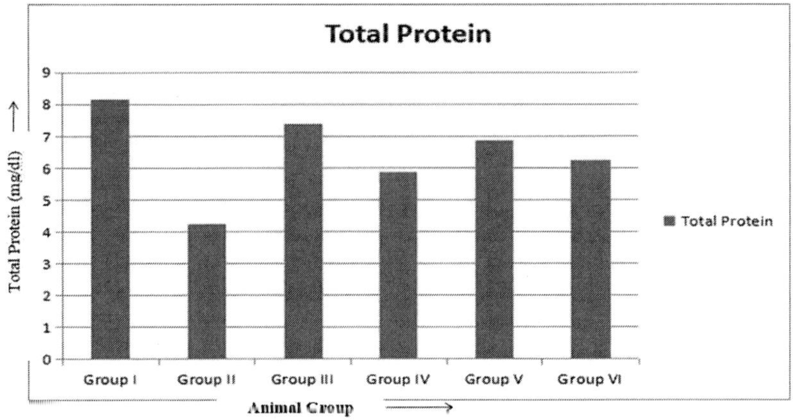

Fig 7-13 Graphical presentation of total protein

Discussion:

The biochemical parameters such as SGPT and SGOT bilirubin, cholesterol, ALP, and total protein of the plant *Ardisia humilis* Vahl were determined. The methanolic extract of *Ardisia humilis* Vahl leaves was administered in three different doses (300, 500, and 700 mg/kg). CCl_4 was used as a hepatotoxic agent. Administration of CCl_4-produced hepatotoxicity showed a significant increase in the serum levels of SGPT,

SGOT, ALP, and bilirubin, and the levels of cholesterol and total protein decreased as compared to the control group. The methanolic extract of *Ardisia humilis* Vahl showed a significant decrease in the serum enzymes SGPT, SGOT, ALP, and bilirubin as compared to the control group. Based on the results obtained, it can be concluded that the methanolic extract of *Ardisia humilis* Vahl leaves seems to induce hepatoprotective activity in rats.

7.8.3 Liver Enzyme Activity

The effects of different doses of methanolic extract of the leaves on the liver enzyme activity of Glutathione and Catalase were determined in the carbon tetrachloride-induced albino rats using Silymarin as a standard drug. The results are summarized in Table 7-12.

Table 7-16 Effects of methanolic extract of *Ardisia humilis* Vahl on Glutathione and Catalase activity levels in experimental animals.

Group	Glutathione (U/mg protein) (mean±SD)	Catalase (U/mg protein) (mean±SD)
G-I Vehicle Control	16.94 ± 0.237	21.47 ± 21.220
G-II Hepatic Control	5.766 ± 0.063	9.71 ± 9.560
G-III Standard Drug	14.58 ± 0.222	19.46 ± 19.260
G-IV Test 1 (300mg/kg)	7.44 ± 0.109	9.87 ± 9.780
G-V Test 2 (500mg/kg)	11.36 ± 0.210	15.95 ±15.670
G-VI Test 3 (700mg/kg)	9.62 ± 0.098	14.26 ± 14.130

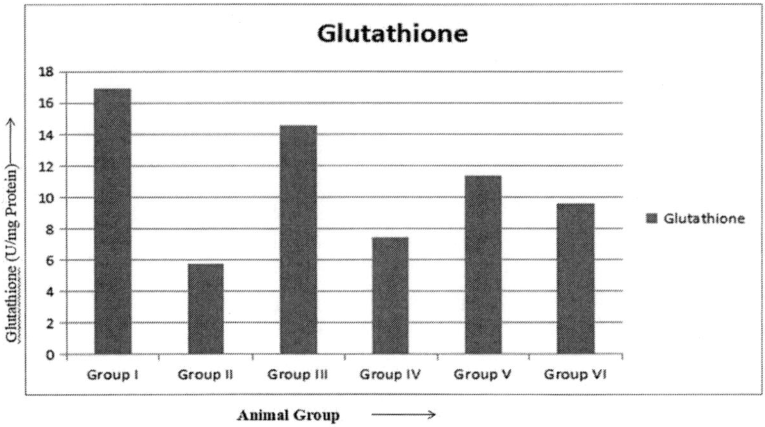

Fig 7-14 Graphical presentation of Glutathione activity

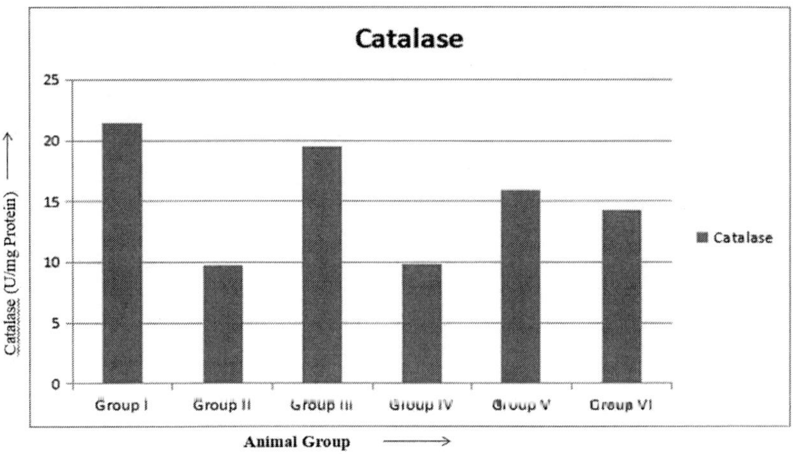

Fig 7-15 Graphical presentation of catalase activity

Discussion:

Liver enzyme parameters (glutathion and catalase) were studied. On the administration of *Ardisia humilis* Vahl methanolic extract, catalase and glutathion levels significantly increased as compared to the control group, and the MEAH (500 mg/kg) showed the highest increasing level of catalase and glutathion as compared to the other two plant extracts (300 and 700 mg/kg). Based on the results obtained, the methanolic extract of *Ardisia humilis* Vahl has a good effect as a hepatoprotective agent.

7.9 Histopathological Examination

The livers were dissected from animals belonging to different groups after sacrificing them. The liver samples were subjected to histopathological examination after carefully performing the processes of alcoholic dehydration, paraffin block embedding, staining, and cutting sections in a microtome as per the procedures described in Section 6.15.4.

The histopathological observations are systematically arranged in Fig 7–16.

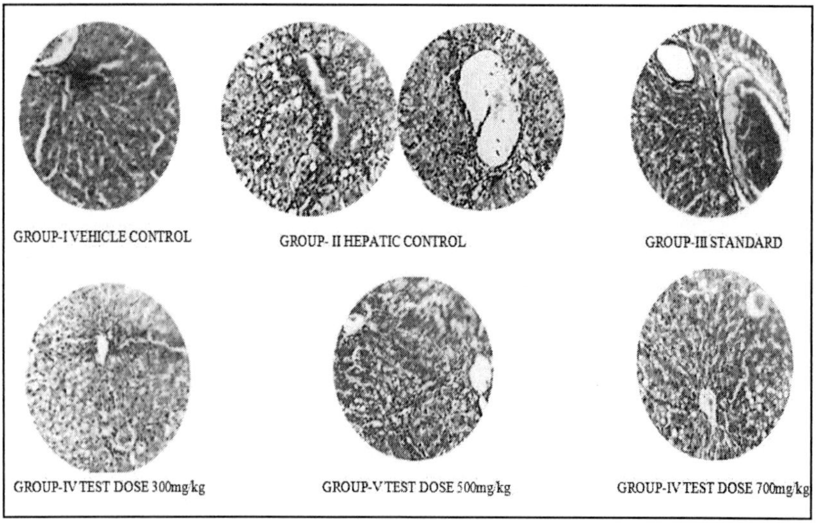

Fig 7-16 Liver sections of the experimental animals. Group-I Vehicle control, Group-II Hepatic control, Group-III Standard Drug, Group-IV Test dose (300mg/kg), Group-V Test dose (500mg/kg), Group-VI Test dose (700mg/kg)

Discussion:

The histopathological studies show the prominent activity of *Ardisia humilis* Vahl leaf extract on CCl_4-induced rats.

- Group I Vehicle Control: shows the normal control liver section of the rat containing the central vein, the portal vein, the hepatocytes, the kupffer cells, and the sinusoids.
- Group II toxic control: toxic control showing distorted central vein, damaged portal vein, no sinusoids, formation of microvacuoles, and less visible hepatocytes
- Group III Standard: Standard treated, showing normal features of the tissues section with a few microvacuolizations, cell death, and congestion in the portal vein.
- Group IV Treated with 300 mg/kg body weight of *Ardisia humilis* Vahl, showing portal vein, some cell death, a few sinusoids, microvacuoles, and a damaged central vein.
- Group V Treated with 500 mg/kg body weight, showing better portal vein and central vein, less cell death, and improved sinusoids.
- Group VI Treated with 700 mg/kg body weight showed improved features compared to other test groups, i.e., fewer hepatocyte deaths and fewer small vacuoles. The sinusoids are very visible with Kuffer cells.

8

SUMMARY AND CONCLUSION

BIMAN BHUYAN AND JENTINOCHET AMRI

Summary of Findings

In-depth reports on pharmacognostic, phytochemical, and pharmacological investigations have been done on the plant *Ardisia humilis* Vahl.

The plant's correct identification for further research has been made possible by the pharmacognostic and phytochemical investigations. To justify and authenticate the drug, morphological, microscopic, and physiochemical characteristics can also be considered as identifying parameters.

The phytoconstituents of various *Ardisia humilis* Vahl extracts would be beneficial in the treatment of many ailments, and the fluorescence examination of powdered drugs is crucial in determining the quality and purity of the drug.

Utilizing the DPPH scavenging, nitric oxide scavenging, and hydroxyl radical scavenging methods, the antioxidant activity of the plant *Ardisia humilis* Vahl was assessed. When compared to standard drugs, the plant extract demonstrated considerable antioxidant activity. This may be the justification for the use of plant extracts in traditional medicine. The chemical makeup and structural characteristics of the active extract components have a significant role in determining the effectiveness of natural antioxidants.

Swiss albino mice were used in acute toxicity trials, and adverse responses were not seen up to dosages of 2000 mg/kg for 48 hours.

Biochemical indices and histology were found to be protective against CCl_4-induced hepatotoxicity throughout 14 days of *in vivo* hepatoprotective activities. According to the findings, Silymarin is more powerful than the methanolic extract of *Ardisia humilis* Vahl. 500 mg/kg and 700 mg/kg doses were found to be more effective than 300 mg/kg body weight.

So, based on the data gathered, it can be stated that the methanolic extract of *Ardisia humilis* Vahl. has hepatoprotective action. This finding appears to validate the plant's traditional usage in hepatoprotection.

More research is needed to uncover the bioactive phytoconstituents found in the crude extracts of this plant and to produce herbal formulations for the treatment of liver disorders.

BIBLIOGRAPHY

Aggarwal, Annu and Bhatt Mohit. 2018. "Advances in treatment of Wilson disease." *Tremor and Other Hyperkinetic Movements* 8:1-13.

Akerele, Olubanke. 1993."Summary of WHO guidelines for the assessment of herbal medicines." *Herbal gram* 28(13): 9-13.

Akinloye, Oluseyi Adeboye, Moshood Olajire Olaniyi. 2011. "Hepatoprotective effect of *Cajanus cajan* on tissue defence system in D-galactosamine-induced hepatitis in rats." *Turkish Journal of Biochemistry/Turk Biyokimya Dergisi,* 36(3):237-241.

Ali, Muhammad, Tariq Khan, Kaneez Fatima, Qurat ul Ain Ali, Muhammad Ovais, Ali Talha Khalil, Ikram Ullah, Abida Raza, Zabta Khan Shinwari, and Muhammad Idrees. 2018. "Selected hepatoprotective herbal medicines: Evidence from ethnomedicinal applications, animal models, and possible mechanism of actions." *Phytotherapy Research*, 32(2): 199-215.

Andrade, Raúl J., and Paul M. Tulkens. 2011."Hepatic safety of antibiotics used in primary care." *Journal of Antimicrobial Chemotherapy*, 66(7): 1431-1446.

Andrade, Raúl J., Mercedes Robles, Eugenia Ulzurrun, M. Isabel Lucena. 2009."Drug-induced liver injury: insights from genetic studies." *Pharmacogenomics,* 10(9): 1467-1487.

Anonymous, Botanical Survey of India. 2007; 1: 235,288,340.

Atmakuri, Lakshmana Rao and Dathi, Suneetha. 2010." Current Trends in Herbal Medicines." *Journal of Pharmacy Research,* 3(1): 109-113.

Awang, Dennis VC. 1997 "Quality control and good manufacturing practices: Safety and efficacy of commercial herbals." *Food and Drug Law Journal*, 52(3): 341-344.

Basha, Jamal, Murthy, Srinivas., C. Prakash, A. Kirthi, K. C. Anuradha. 2016. "Pharmacognostical standardization, preliminary phytochemical investigation of root stocks of *Ardisia solanacea* Roxb." *Journal of Chemical and Pharmaceutical Research,* 8(8): 1107-1113.

Bedi, Onkar, Reddy Krishna, V. Bijjem, Kumar Puneet, Gauttam Vinod. 2016. "Herbal Induced Hepatoprotection and Hepatotoxicity: A Critical Review." *Indian Journal of Physiology and Pharmacology,* 60(1): 6-21.

Begriche, Karima, Laetitia Knockaert, Julie Massart, Marie-Anne Robin, Bernard Fromenty. 2009. "Mitochondrial dysfunction in nonalcoholic steatohepatitis (NASH): are there drugs able to improve it?" *Drug Discovery Today: Disease Mechanisms,* 6(1-4): e11-e23.

Bell, Lauren N., and Chalasani Naga. 2009."Epidemiology of idiosyncratic drug-induced liver injury." In *Seminars in Liver Disease,* 29(4):337-347.

Binduja, Saraswat, Visen P. K. S., Dayal R., Agarwal D. P., Patnaik G. K. 1996."Protective action of ursolic acid against chemical induced hepato-toxicity in rats."*Indian Journal of Pharmacology,* 28(4): 232.

Bissell, D. Montgomery, Gregory J. Gores, Debra L. Laskin, Jay H. Hoofnagle. 2001."Drug-induced liver injury: mechanisms and test systems." *Hepatology,* 33(4): 1009-1013.

Bradbury, P., K. C. Gordon, J. D. Bancroft, A. Stevens. 1990. "Theory and practice of histological techniques." *Connective tissue and stains,* 119-42. Edinburgh London Melbourne and New York: Churchill Livingstone Inc.

Bruno, Savino, Patrick Maisonneuve, Paola Castellana, Nicole Rotmensz, Sonia Rossi, Marco Maggioni, Marcello Persico. 2005. "Incidence and risk factors for non-alcoholic steatohepatitis: prospective study of 5408 women enrolled in Italian tamoxifen chemoprevention trial." *BMJ,* 330(7497): 932.

Cahill, Alan, Carol C. Cunningham, Masayuki Adachi, Hiromasa Ishii, Shannon M. Bailey, Bernard Fromenty, Adrian Davies. 2002. "Effects of alcohol and oxidative stress on liver pathology: the role of the mitochondrion." *Alcoholism: Clinical and Experimental Research,* 26(6): 907-915.

Chalasani, Naga, and Einar Björnsson. 2010."Risk factors for idiosyncratic drug-induced liver injury." *Gastroenterology,* 138(7): 2246-2259.

Chattopadhyay, Rabi Ranjan, and Bhattacharyya, Sabyasachi. 2007. "*Terminalia chebula*: An update." *Pharmacognosy Reviews,* 1(1):151-156.

Chieli, Elisabetta and Gino Malvaldi. 1984. "Role of the microsomal FAD-containing monooxygenase in the liver toxicity of thioacetamide S-oxide." *Toxicology,* 31(1): 41-52.

Coghlan ME, Sommadossi JP, Jhala NC, Many WJ, Saag MS, Johnson VA. 2001. Symptomatic lactic acidosis in hospitalized antiretroviral-treated patients with human immunodeficiency virus infection, a report of 12 cases, Clin Infect Dis. 33(11): 1914-1921.

Colegate, Steven M, and Molyneux, Russell J. 2008. *Bioactive Natural*

Products: Detection, Isolation and Structural Determination. New York: CRC Press.

Daly, Ann K., and Chris P. Day. 2009. "Genetic association studies in drug-induced liver injury." *Seminars in Liver Disease*, 29(4):400-411.

Danan, Gaby, Bernuau, Jacques Raymond, Claude, Degott Gérard, Babanyand Benhamou, Jean Pierre. 1985."Pirprofen-induced fulminant hepatitis." *Gastroenterology,* 89(1): 210-213.

Dawkins, M. J. R. 1963. "Carbon tetrachloride poisoning in the liver of the new-born rat." *The Journal of Pathology and Bacteriology,* 85(1): 189-196.

De Smet, Peter AGM. 1997. "The role of plant-derived drugs and herbal medicines in healthcare." *Drugs,* 54(6): 801-840.

Demeilliers, Christine, Caroline Maisonneuve, Alain Grodet, Abdellah Mansouri, Richard Nguyen, Marina Tinel, Philippe Lettéron. 2002. "Impaired adaptive resynthesis and prolonged depletion of hepatic mitochondrial DNA after repeated alcohol binges in mice." *Gastroenterology,* 123(4): 1278-1290.

Doumas, Basil T. 1975. "Standards for total serum protein assays—a collaborative study." *Clinical chemistry.* 21(8): 1159-1166.

Dubey, N. K., Kumar Rajesh, and Tripathi Pramila. 2004. "Global Promotion of Herbal Medicine: India's Opportunity." *Current Science,* 86(1): 37–41.

Eidi, Akram, Pejman Mortazavi, Maryam Bazargan, Jalal Zaringhalam. 2012."Hepatoprotective activity of cinnamon ethanolic extract against CCI4-induced liver injury in rats." *Excli Journal*, 11: 495-507.

Ekstedt, Mattias, Lennart E. Franzén, Ulrik L. Mathiesen, Holmqvist Marika, Göran Bodemar, Stergios Kechagias. 2007."Statins in non-alcoholic fatty liver disease and chronically elevated liver enzymes: a histopathological follow-up study." *Journal of Hepatology,* 47(1): 135-141.

Evans, William Charles. 2009. *Trease and Evans' Pharmacognosy.* UK:W.B Saunders, Elsevier Health Sciences.

Fabbrini, Elisa, Shelby Sullivan, Samuel Klein. 2010. "Obesity and nonalcoholic fatty liver disease: biochemical, metabolic, and clinical implications." *Hepatology,* 51(2): 679-689.

Fernandez, Felix G., John Ritter, J. Wendell Goodwin, David C. Linehan, William G. Hawkins, Steven M. Strasberg. 2005. "Effect of steatohepatitis associated with irinotecan or oxaliplatin pretreatment on resectability of hepatic colorectal metastases." *Journal of the American College of Surgeons,* 200(6): 845-853.

Fromenty, B., M. A. Robin, A. Igoudjil, A. Igoudjil, D. Pessayre. 2004."The ins and outs of mitochondrial dysfunction in NASH." *Diabetes &Metabolism,* 30(2): 121-138.

Fulda, Simone, Lorenzo Galluzzi, Guido Kroemer. 2010."Targeting mitochondria for cancer therapy." *Nature reviews Drug Discovery,* 9(6): 447-464.

García-Ruiz, Inmaculada, Rodríguez-Juan Cristina, Teresa Díaz-Sanjuán, Martínez Miguel Ángel, Teresa Muñoz-Yagüe, José A. Solís-Herruzo. 2007. "Effects of rosiglitazone on the liver histology and mitochondrial function in ob/ob mice." *Hepatology,* 46(2): 414-423.

Gossell-Williams, M., R. E. Simon, M. E. West. 2006. "The past and present use of plants for medicines." *West Indian Medical Journal,* 55(4): 217-218.

Government of India, Ministry of AYUSH. 2016. *The Ayurvedic Pharmacopoeia of India.* Ghaziabad: Pharmacopoeia Commission for Indian Medicine & Homoeopathy.

Gulati, Kavita., Reshi, Mohd Rafi, Rai, Nishant, Ray, Arunabha. 2018. "Hepatotoxicity: Its mechanisms, experimental evaluation and protective strategies." *American Journal of Pharmacology,* 1 (1): 1004.

Güldütuna, Sükrettin, Guido Zimmer, Matthias Imhof, Bhatti, Susan Tiangeng You, Ulrich Leuschner. 1993. "Molecular aspects of membrane stabilization by ursodeoxycholate." *Gastroenterology,* 104(6): 1736-1744.

Gupta, M. K., Sharma, P. K., Ansari, S. H., Lagarkha, R. 2006. "Pharmacognostical evaluation of *Grewiaasiatica* fruits."*International Journal of Plant Science,* 1(2): 249-251.

Hagey, Lee R., Crombie,Diane L. Edgard Espinosa, Martin C. Carey, HirotsuneIgimi, Alan F. Hofmann. 1993. "Ursodeoxycholic acid in the Ursidae: biliary bile acids of bears, pandas, and related carnivores." *Journal of Lipid Research,* 34(11): 1911-1917.

Harbrone, Jeffrey B. 2012. *Phytochemical Methods A Guide To Modern Techniques of Plant Analysis.*Netherlands: Springer.

Hautekeete, M. L., C. Degott, J-P. Benhamou. 1990. "Microvesicular steatosis of the liver." *Acta Clinica Belgica,* 45(5): 311-326.

Hussain, Zulfia, Junaid Ali Khan, Arfa Arshad, Palwasha Asif, Haroon Rashid, Muhammad Imran Arshad. 2019. "Protective effects of *Cinnamomum zeylanicum* L.(Dalchini) in acetaminophen-induced oxidative stress, hepatotoxicity and nephrotoxicity in mouse model." *Biomedicine & Pharmacotherapy,* 109: 2285-2292.

Jones, Dean P., Lemasters, John J. Derick Han, Urs A. Boelsterli, Neil Kaplowitz. 2010. "Mechanisms of pathogenesis in drug hepatotoxicity putting the stress on mitochondria." *Molecular Interventions,* 10(2): 98.

Joshi, Nirali, and M. Shankar. 2016."Global market analysis of herbal drug formulations." *International Journal of Ayurveda and Pharmaceutical Chemistry*, 4(1): 59-65.

Kamboj, Ved Prakash. 2000. "Herbal medicine". *Current Science*, 78 (1): 35-39.

Kaplan, Lawrence A., Amadeo J. Pesce, Amin A. Mohammad, Ewa A. Filipowicz. 1998. "Clinical Chemistry: Theory, Analysis, and Correlation." *Archives of Pathology and Laboratory Medicine.* 122(8): 752-757.

Kaplowitz, Neil. (2007). "Immunological Mechanisms in Drug-Induced Liver Injury" In Drug *Induced Liver Disease*, edited by Neil. Kaplowitz, and Laurie DeLeve, 334-348. Philadephia:CRC Press.

Kashaw, Varsha, Nema Amit K., Agarwal Abhinav. 2011. "Hepatoprotective prospective of herbal drugs and their vesicular carriers–a review." *International Journal of Research in Pharmaceutical and Biomedical Sciences,* 2(2): 360-374.

Keppler, Dietrich, Jürgen Pausch, Karl Decker. 1974."Selective uridine triphosphate deficiency induced by D-galactosamine in liver and reversed by pyrimidine nucleotide precursors: effect on ribonucleic acid synthesis." *Journal of Biological Chemistry,* 249(1): 211-216.

Ketcham, Stephanie A., Ashraf Muhammad, Madhavarao Chikkathur N. 2017. "Direct quantification of protein glycan phosphorylation." *BioTechniques.* 63(3): 117-123.

Khandelwal, Kishanchandra Radhesyam. 2004. *Practical Pharmacognosy-Techniques and Experiments*.Pune:NiraliPrakashan.

Khatun, Amina, Mahmudur Rahman, Sumaiya Kabir, Md Nahid Akter, Sadia Afreen Chowdhury. 2013. "Phytochemical and pharmacological properties of methanolic extract of *Ardisia humilis* Vahl. (Myrsinaceae)."*International Journal of Research in Ayurveda and Pharmacy,* 4(1): 38-41.

Khatun, Amina, Rahman Mahmudur, Kabir Sumaiya, Akter Nahid, Chowdhury Sadia Afreen.2013. "Phytochemical and pharmacological properties of methanolic extract of *Ardisia humilis* Vahl. (Myrsinaceae). "*International Journal of Research in Ayurveda and Pharmacy,* 4(1): 38-41.

Kleiner, David E., Gaffey Michael J., Sallie Richard, Tsokos Maria, Larry Nichols, Robin McKenzie, Stephen E. Straus, Jay H. Hoofnagle. 1997. "Histopathologic changes associated with fialuridine hepatotoxicity."

Modern Pathology: An Official Journal of the United States and Canadian Academy of Pathology, Inc, 10(3): 192-199.

Kokate, Chandra Kant. 2006. *Practical Pharmacognosy*. Delhi: Vallabh Prakashan.

Kokoshi, Charles J.,Kokoshi, Robert J,SlamaFrank J. 1958. "Fluorescence of powdered vegetable drugs under ultraviolet radiations."*Journal of Pharmaceutical Sciences.* 47: 715-717.

Kumar, Vadlapudi and V. Kumar. 2009. "An overview of herbal medicine." *International Journal of Pharmaceutical Sciences*, 1(1): 1-20.

Kwon, Jae-Woo, Shin Eun-Soon, Jong-Eun Lee, Sang-Heon Kim, Sang-Hoon Kim, Young-Koo Jee, Yoon-Keun Kim, Hae-Sim Park, Kyung-Up Min, Heung-Woo Park. 2012. "Genetic variations in TXNRD1 as potential predictors of drug-induced liver injury." *Allergy, Asthma & Immunology Research,* 4(3): 132-136.

Larrey, Dominique.2002."Epidemiology and individual susceptibility to adverse drug reactions affecting the liver." In *Seminars in Liver Disease*, 22(2):145-156.

Lauressergues, Emilie, Bart Staels, Karine Valeille, Zouher Majd, Dean W. Hum, Patrick Duriez, Didier Cussac. 2010. "Antipsychotic drug action on SREBPs-related lipogenesis and cholesterogenesis in primary rat hepatocytes." *Naunyn-Schmiedeberg's Archives of Pharmacology,* 381(5): 427-439.

Lazarou, Jason, Bruce H. Pomeranz, Paul N. Corey.1998. "Incidence of adverse drug reactions in hospitalized patients: a meta-analysis of prospective studies." *Journal of the American Medical Association*, 279(15): 1200-1205.

Le Bricquir, Yann, Dominique Larrey, Pierre Blanc, Georges Philippe Pageaux, Henri Michel. 1994. "Tianeptine—an instance of drug-induced hepatotoxicity predicted by prospective experimental studies." *Journal of Hepatology,* 21(5): 771-773.

Lillie, RalphDougall. 1965. *Histopathologic Technique and Practical Histochemistry*. New York: McGraw Hill Book Co.

Lucena, M. Isabel, Raúl J. Andrade, Fernández M. Carmen, Pachkoria Ketevan, Gloria Pelaez, José A. Durán, Macarena Villar. 2006. "Determinants of the clinical expression of amoxicillin-clavulanate hepatotoxicity: a prospective series from Spain." *Hepatology,* 44(4): 850-856.

Magielse, Joanna, Teresita Arcoraci, Annelies Breynaert, Ines van Dooren, Cimanga Kanyanga, Erik Fransen, Viviane Van Hoof. 2013. "Antihepatotoxic activity of a quantified Desmodium adscendens decoction and D-pinitol against chemically-induced liver damage in rats." *Journal of Ethnopharmacology,* 146(1): 250-256.

Malhi, Harmeet, Gregory J. Gores, Lemasters John J. 2006. "Apoptosis and necrosis in the liver: a tale of two deaths?" *Hepatology,* 43(S1): S31-S44.

Mallhi, Tauqeer Hussain, M. Qadir, Yusra Habib Khan, Muhammad Ali. "Hepatoprotective activity of aqueous methanolic extract of Morusnigra against paracetamol-induced hepatotoxicity in mice." *Bangladesh Journal of Pharmacology* 9 (2014): 60-66.

Masubuchi, Yasuhiro, Chieko Suda, Toshiharu Horie. 2005. "Involvement of mitochondrial permeability transition in acetaminophen-induced liver injury in mice." *Journal of Hepatology,*42(1): 110-116.

McQuaid, Albert, Lamand Michel, Mason James. 1992. "The interactions of penicillamine with copper in vivo and the effect on hepatic metallothionein levels and copper/zinc distribution: the implications for Wilson's disease and arthritis therapy." *The Journal of laboratory and clinical medicine* 119(6): 744-750.

Meagher E, Thomson C. 1999. "Vitamin and Mineral Therapy." In *Medical Nutrition and Disease*, Edited by G Morrison and L Hark, Malden, 105-114. Massachusetts: Blackwell Science Inc.

Mukherjee, Pulok Kumar. 2002.*Quality Control of Herbal Drugs – An Approach to Evaluation of Botanicals.* New Delhi:Business Horizon Pharmaceutical Publisher

Naik, G. H., Priyadarsini, K. I., Satav, Jagannath G., Banavalikar, M. M., Sohoni,D. P., Biyani, M. K., Mohana, H. 2003. "Comparative antioxidant activity of individual herbal components used in Ayurvedic medicine."*Phytochemistry,* 63(1): 97-104.

Nanashima Kazutaka, Mawatari Tsutomu, Tahara Naoko, Higuchi Norihide, Nakaura Ayano, Tatsuo Inamine, Kondo Shinji, Yanagihara Katsunori, Fukushima Kiyoyasu, Suyama Naofumi, Kohno Shigeru, Tsukamoto Kazuhiro. 2012."Genetic variants in antioxidant pathway: risk factors for hepatotoxicity in tuberculosis patients." *Tuberculosis,* 92(3): 253-259.

Nayak, B. Shivananda, Julien R. Marshall, Godwin Isitor, Andrew Adogwa.2011. "Hypoglycemic and hepatoprotective activity of fermented fruit juice of *Morinda citrifolia* (Noni) in diabetic rats." *Evidence-Based Complementary and Alternative Medicine,* 2011:1-5

Oliver, Daniel. 1994. *Study of Indian Botany.* New Delhi: Atlantic Publishers.

Ostapowicz, George, Fontana J.Robert, Schiødt V. Frank, Larson Anne, Timothy J. Davern, Steven HB Han, Timothy M. McCashland. 2002.

"Results of a prospective study of acute liver failure at 17 tertiary care centers in the United States." *Annals of Internal Medicine,* 137(12): 947-954.

Ottolenghi, Athos. 1959."Interaction of ascorbic acid and mitochondrial lipides." *Archives of Biochemistry and Biophysics,* 79: 355-363.

Owais, Mohammad, Ahmad, Iqbal, Khan,Shazia, Khan, Umber, Ahmad, Nadeem.2006. "An Alternative Holistic Medicinal Approach to the Total Management of Hepatic Disorders: A Novel Polyherbal Formulation." In *Modern Phytomedicine, Turning Medicinal Plants into Drugs*, edited by Iqbal Ahmad, Farrukh Aqil, and Mohammad Owais, 233-245. Weinheim: WILEY-VCH Verlag GmbH & Co.

Pande, Jitendra Nath, Singh Sivaram Prasad, Khilnani Gopi Chand, KhilnaniS., Tandon Rakesh Kumar. 1996. "Risk factors for hepatotoxicity from antituberculosis drugs: a case-control study." *Thorax,* 51(2): 132-136.

Paramesha, Mahadevappa, Chapeyil K. Ramesh, Venkatarangaiah Krishna, Yelegara S. Ravi Kumar, Karur MM Parvathi. 2011. "Hepatoprotective and in vitro antioxidant effect of *Carthamus tinctorious* L, var Annigeri-2-, an oil-yielding crop, against CCl_4-induced liver injury in rats." *Pharmacognosy magazine,* 7(28): 289-297.

Paumgartner, Gustav, Ulrich Beuers. 2002. "Ursodeoxycholic acid in cholestatic liver disease: mechanisms of action and therapeutic use revisited." *Hepatology,* 36(3): 525-531.

Pessayre, Dominique, Abdellah Mansouri, Berson Alain, Fromenty Bernard. 2010. "Mitochondrial Involvement in Drug-Induced Liver Injury". In *Adverse Drug Reactions: Handbook of Experimental Pharmacology,* edited by Uetrecht, J.,311-365. Berlin:Springer.

Pessayre, Dominique, Delphine Haouzi, FauDaniel, Marie Anne Robin, Abdellah Mansouri, Alain Berson. 1999."Withdrawal of life support, altruistic suicide, fratricidal killing and euthanasia by lymphocytes: different forms of drug-induced hepatic apoptosis." *Journal of Hepatology*, 31(4): 760-770.

Pugliese, Michela, Vito Biondi, Enrico Gugliandolo, Patrizia Licata, Alessio Filippo Peritore, Rosalia Crupi, and Annamaria Passantino. 2021. "D-Penicillamine: The state of the art in humans and in dogs from a Pharmacological and regulatory perspective." *Antibiotics* 10 (6): 648.

Quattroachi, Umberto. 2012. *CRC World Dictionary of Medicinal and Poisonous Plants.* Boca Raton: CRC Press.

Raina, M.K.2003. “Quality Control of Herbal and Herbo-Mineral Formulations.”*Indian Journal of Natural Products*, 19:11-15.

Ramadori, G., F. Moriconi, I. Moriconi, J. Dudas. 2008. "Physiology and Pathophysiology of Liver Inflammation, Damage and Repair." *Journal of Physiology and Pharmacology*, 59: 107-117.

Ramappa, Vidyasagar, Guruprasad P. Aithal.2013. "Hepatotoxicity related to anti-tuberculosis drugs: mechanisms and management." *Journal of Clinical and Experimental Hepatology,* 3(1): 37-49.

Randhawa, GS, and Mukhopadhyay, Amithabha. 2010. *Floriculture in India.* New Delhi: Allied Publisher.

Rane, Jesika, R. Jadhao, R. L. Bakal. 2016."Liver diseases and herbal drugs-A review." *Journal of Innovations in Pharmaceutical and Biological Sciences*, 3(2): 24-36.

Rosenberg, Peter, Urwitz Hanna, Johannesson Anders, Ros Anne-Marie, Lindholm Johan, Nils Kinnman, Rolf Hultcrantz. 2007."Psoriasis patients with diabetes type 2 are at high risk of developing liver fibrosis during methotrexate treatment." *Journal of Hepatology,* 46(6): 1111-1118.

Roy, Chanchal, Kamath, Jagadish., Asad, Mohammed. 2006. “Hepatoprotactive activity of *Psidium guajava* Linn. leaf extract.” *Indian Journal of Experimental Biology,* 44(4): 305-11.

Roy, Saumendu Deb, Das Sumit, Shil Dibyendu, Dutta Koushik Nandan. 2012. "Herbal hepatoprotective agents: a review." *World Journal of Pharmaceutical Research,* 1(2): 87-99.

Ruch, Randall J, Cheng, Shu Jun, Klaunig, James E. 1989. “Prevention of cytotoxicity and inhibition of intercellular communication by antioxidant catechins isolated from Chinese green tea.” *Carcinogenesis*, 10(6):1003-1008.

Saltos, Mariela Beatriz Vera, Blanca Fabiola Naranjo Puente, Luigi Milella, Nunziatina De Tommasi, Fabrizio Dal Piaz, Alessandra Braca. 2015. "Antioxidant and free radical scavenging activity of phenolics from *Bidens humilis*." *Planta médica,* 81(12/13): 1056-1064.

Sanz, Alberto, Pilar Caro, Victoria Ayala, Manuel Portero-Otin, Reinald Pamplona, Gustavo Barja. 2006. "Methionine restriction decreases mitochondrial oxygen radical generation and leak as well as oxidative damage to mitochondrial DNA and proteins." *The FASEB Journal,* 20(8): 1064-1073.

Saphner, Tom, Shirley Triest-Robertson, Hailun Li, Paul Holzman. 2009."The association of nonalcoholic steatohepatitis and tamoxifen in patients with breast cancer." *Cancer: Interdisciplinary International Journal of the American Cancer Society,* 115(14): 3189-3195.

Saumya, SM, Mahaboob, Basha P. 2011. "*In vitro* evaluation of free radical scavenging activities of *Panax ginseng* and *Lagerstroemia speciosa*: a comparative analysis." *International Journal of Pharmacy and Pharmaceutical Sciences*, 3(1):165-169.

Schuetz, Erin G., Stephen Strom, Kazuto Yasuda, Valerie Lecureur, Mahfoud Assem, Cynthia Brimer, Jatinder Lamba. 2001. "Disrupted bile acid homeostasis reveals an unexpected interaction among nuclear hormone receptors, transporters, and cytochrome P450." *Journal of Biological Chemistry,* 276(42): 39411-39418.

Sears, Margaret. 2013. "Chelation: harnessing and enhancing heavy metal detoxification—a review." *The Scientific World Journal* 2013:1-13.

Seifert, Erin L., Carmen Estey, Jian Y. Xuan, Harper Mary-Ellen. 2010. "Electron transport chain-dependent and-independent mechanisms of mitochondrial H_2O_2 emission during long-chain fatty acid oxidation." *Journal of Biological Chemistry,* 285(8): 5748-5758.

Selvam, N. Thamizh, V. Venkatakrishnan, R.Dhamodharan, S. Murugesan, S. Damodar Kumar. 2013."Hepatoprotective activity of methanolic extract of *Syzygium jambos* (Linn.) leaf against paracetamol intoxicated Wistar albino rats." *Ayu* 34(3): 305-308.

Sembulingam, Kirma, and Prema, Sembulingam. 2010. *Essentials of medical physiology*. JP Medical Ltd: New Delhi.

Sengottuvelu, Singaravel, Srinivasan, Duraisamy, Rasalingam, Duraisami, Jothivel, Nadhakumar, Vasudevan, Mani, Thangavel, Sivakumar. 2010. "Hepatoprotective activity of *Trianthema decandra* on CCl_4 induced hepatotoxicity on rats." *International Journal of Green Pharmacy.* 5(4): 122-125.

Shah, Rajal, Parmar,Sachin, Bhatt,Punit, Chanda, Sumitra. 2011. "Evaluation of hepatoprotective activity of ethyl acetate fraction of *Tephrosia purpurea.*" *Pharmacologyonline,* 3: 188-194.

Shankar, Rama, G. S. Lavekar, S. Deb, and B. K. Sharma. 2012. "Traditional healing practice and folk medicines used by Mishing community of North East India." *Journal of Ayurveda and Integrative Medicine,* 3(3): 124.

Shi, Zi-Qi, Song De-Fang, Li Ruo-Qian, Yang Hua, Qi Lian-Wen, Xin Gui-Zhong, Wang Ding-Qian *et al.* 2014. "Identification of effective combinatorial markers for quality standardization of herbal medicines." *Journal of Chromatography, A* 1345: 78-85.

Shivananda Nayak, B., Julien R. Marshall, Godwin Isitor, Adogwa Andrew.2011. "Hypoglycemic and hepatoprotective activity of fermented fruit juice of *Morinda citrifolia* (Noni) in diabetic rats".

Evidence-Based Complementary Alternative Medicine, 2011:1–5.doi:10.1155/2011/875293.

Snijdewind, Ingrid JM, Colette Smit, Mieke H. Godfried, Jeannine FJB Nellen, Frank de Wolf, Kees Boer, Marchina E. van der Ende. 2012."HCV coinfection, an important risk factor for hepatotoxicity in pregnant women starting antiretroviral therapy." *Journal of Infection,* 64(4): 409-416.

Talwani, Rohit, Bruce L. Gilliam, and Charles Howell. 2011."Infectious diseases and the liver." *Clinics in Liver Disease*, 15(1): 111-130.

Tietz, Norbert W. 1995. "Clinical guide to laboratory tests."In *Clinical guide to laboratory tests*, 1096-1106.

Vaidya, Ashok and Thomas Devasagayam. 2007. "Current status of herbal drugs in India: an overview." *Journal of Clinical Biochemistry and Nutrition,* 41(1): 1-11.

Velsor, Leonard W., Kovacevic Miro, Kovacevic Mark, Leitner Heather M., William Lewis, and Brian J. Day. 2004. "Mitochondrial oxidative stress in human hepatoma cells exposed to stavudine." *Toxicology and Applied Pharmacology,* 199(1): 10-19.

Verma, Amita, Mubashir Masoodi, Bahar Ahmed. 2012. "Lead finding from whole plant of *Marrubium vulgare* L. with hepatoprotective potentials through in silico methods." *Asian Pacific Journal of Tropical Biomedicine,* 2(3): S1308-S1311.

Wairt, Christophe. 2006. *Medicinal Plants of Asia and the Pacific.* Boca Raton: CRC Press.

Wallace, Douglas C., Weiwei Fan, Procaccio Vincent. 2010. "Mitochondrial energetics and therapeutics." *Annual Review of Pathology,* 5: 297.

Wallis, Thomas Edward. 2005. *Textbook of Pharmacognosy*. New Delhi: CBS publisher and Distributors.

Wankhar, Wankupar, Sakthivel Srinivasan, Ravindran Rajan, Sheeladevi Rathinasamy. 2015."Phytochemicals screening and antimicrobial efficacy of *Scoparia dulcis* Linn (Scrophulariaceae) against clinical isolates." *Journal of Pharmacognosy and Phytochemistry,* 3(6):17-21.

Weber, Lutz WD, Meinrad Boll, Stampfl Andreas. 2003. "Hepatotoxicity and mechanism of action of haloalkanes: carbon tetrachloride as a toxicological model." *Critical Reviews in Toxicology,* 33(2): 105-136.

Wilke, Russell A., Debbie W. Lin, Dan M. Roden, Watkins Paul B., David Flockhart, Issam Zineh, Kathleen M. Giacomini, and Ronald M. Krauss. 2007. "Identifying genetic risk factors for serious adverse drug reactions: current progress and challenges." *Nature Reviews Drug Discovery,* 6(11): 904-916.

Winslow, Lisa Corbin, and Kroll David J. 1998. "Herbs as medicines." *Archives of Internal Medicine*, 158(20): 2192-2199.

World Health Organization. 1991. Guidelines for the assessment of herbal medicines. No. WHO/TRM/91.4. Unpublished. World Health Organization.

World Health Organization. 1998. *Quality Control Methods for Medicinal Plant Materials*. Geneva:World Health Organization.

Wu, Zheng-yi, Ihsan A. 1996.*Flora of China-Myrsinaceae through Loganiaceae: [Hauptbd.]*. Beijing:Science Press.

Yang, Li-Hung, Tzer-Ming Chen, Sung-Tsai Yu, Yen-Hui Chen. 2007. "Olanzapine induces SREBP-1-related adipogenesis in 3T3-L1 cells." *Pharmacological Research,* 56(3): 202-208.

Zimmerman, Hyman J. 1999. *Hepatotoxicity: The Adverse Effects of Drugs and other Chemicals on the Liver*.Philadelphia:Lippincot Williams.